Prevention of Nausea and Vomiting in Cancer Patients

Development of this book was supported by funding from Helsinn

Prevention of Nausea and Vomiting in Cancer Patients

Matti Aapro
Multidisciplinary Oncology Institute
Clinique de Genolier
Genolier
Vaud, Switzerland

Karin Jordan
Clinic for Internal Medicine
Department of Oncology/ Hematology
Martin Luther University Hospital
Halle-Wittenberg
Halle, Germany

Petra Feyer
Department of Radio-oncology and Nuclear Medicine
Vivantes Clinics
Berlin-Neukölln
Berlin, Germany

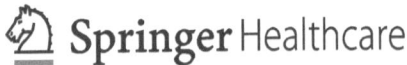

Springer Healthcare

Published by Springer Healthcare Ltd, 236 Gray's Inn Road, London, WC1X 8HB, UK.

www.springerhealthcare.com

British Library Cataloguing-in-Publication Data.

A catalogue record for this book is available from the British Library.

ISBN 978-1-908517-87-6

Although every effort has been made to ensure that drug doses and other information are presented accurately in this publication, the ultimate responsibility rests with the prescribing physician. Neither the publisher nor the authors can be held responsible for errors or for any consequences arising from the use of the information contained herein. Any product mentioned in this publication should be used in accordance with the prescribing information prepared by the manufacturers. No claims or endorsements are made for any drug or compound at present under clinical investigation.

Project editor: Alla Zarifyan
Designer: Joe Harvey
Artworker: Sissan Mollerfors
Production: Marina Maher

Contents

Author biographies   vii

1 Introduction   **1**

Antiemetic agents   1

History of antiemetic therapy   2

References   3

2 Pathophysiology and classification of chemotherapy-induced nausea and vomiting   **5**

Historical background   5

Mechanisms of chemotheraphy-induced nausea and vomiting   6

Neurotransmitters   8

Classification of nausea and vomiting   13

References   14

3 Risk factors associated with nausea and vomiting after chemotherapy   **15**

Emetogenic potential of chemotherapy   15

Patient risk factors   17

References   19

4 Risk factors associated with nausea and vomiting a fter radiotherapy   **21**

Classification of radiotherapy-induced nausea and vomiting   21

References   22

5 Antiemetic drugs   **23**

Serotonin receptor antagonists   23

Steroids   27

Neurokinin-1 receptor antagonists   28

Dopamine receptor antagonists   29

Olanzapine   30

Cannabinoids   31

Benzodiazepines   31

Antihistamines   31

Herbs as antiemetics   32

References   32

**6 Antiemetic prophylaxis of chemotherapy-induced nausea
     and vomiting   37**

Prevention of acute nausea and emesis (within the first 24 hours of

   chemotherapy treatment)   39

Prevention of delayed nausea and emesis

   (days 2–5 after chemotherapy)   39

Therapy against anticipatory nausea and vomiting   40

Therapy in cases of insufficient antiemetic efficacy   41

Multiday chemotherapy   42

High-dose chemotherapy   42

References   42

**7 Antiemetic prophylaxis of radiotherapy-induced nausea
     and vomiting   45**

Antiemetics and their efficacy for radiotherapy-induced nausea and vomiting

                                                               46

Guideline-based prophylaxis and treatment of radiotherapy-induced nausea

   and vomiting   50

References   52

**8 Summary of the approach to treatment of chemotherapy-
     induced nausea and vomiting   55**

References   57

9 Conclusions and future directions   59

Author biographies

Matti Aapro, MD received his medical degree from the Faculty of Medicine, University of Geneva, Switzerland. He was subsequently a fellow at the Arizona Cancer Center in Tucson, USA, and later was the founding chair of the Medical and Radiation Therapy Department at the European Institute of Oncology in Milan, Italy.

He is presently the dean of the Multidisciplinary Oncology Institute, Genolier, Switzerland. Dr Aapro serves as Executive Director of the International Society for Geriatric Oncology. He was a member of the Board of the European Organization for Research and Treatment of Cancer. Dr Aapro is a board member and a past-president of the Multinational Association for Supportive Care in Cancer (MASCC).

Dr Aapro chaired the scientific and organizing committees of the International Union Against Cancer (UICC) World Cancer Congress (WCC) of 2008 and continues to serve UICC for the WCC in China in 2010. He is a member of the European Cancer Organisation/European Society of Medical Oncology (ECCO/ESMO) 2011 Scientific Committee. He coordinates the Sharing Progress in Cancer Care program of the European School of Oncology. Dr Aapro is the editor-in-chief of *Critical Reviews in Oncology/Hematology*, as well as the associate editor of *Annals of Oncology*, the associate editor for the geriatric section of *The Oncologist* and member of the editorial board of *Journal of Clinical Oncology* (breast section). He has authored more than 300 publications and his major interests are new drug development, breast cancer, cancer in the elderly, and supportive care.

Karin Jordan, MD, PhD graduated from Martin Luther University of Halle-Wittenberg, Germany, after internships in the bone-marrow transplantation program at the University of California, San Diego, USA, and in general surgery at the University of Newcastle, UK. Following a number of posts at the University Hospital, Halle, and Bernward Hospital, Hildesheim, Germany, she was appointed as a specialist in internal medicine in 2007 and is now an associate professor of Medical Oncology and Supportive Care in the Department of Oncology/Haematology, University Hospital, Halle. She has been the vice executive director of the ethics committee at the University of Halle since 2009.

Dr Jordan has served as a board member of the ESMO Consensus Panel 2008 on the treatment of testicular cancer, the Multinational Association of Supportive Care in Cancer MASCC/ESMO Antiemetic Guideline Consensus Panel 2009 in Perugia, Italy, and the German Cancer Society Consensus Panel on paravasation induced by cytotoxic agents. She holds the cochair of Supportive Care within the German Society of Medical Oncology and is the associate chair of the German Association of Supportive Care in Oncology, Rehabilitation and Social Medicine. She is a member of a number of national and international hematology and oncology societies.

Dr Jordan has authored and coauthored more than 70 articles in national and international journals. Her principal area of interest is supportive care with a special focus on antiemetic treatment of chemotherapy-induced nausea and vomiting and side effects of new drugs. Further major interests are sarcoma and testicular cancer.

Petra Feyer, MD, PhD studied medicine at the Universities of Sofia, Bulgaria and Leipzig, Germany. At the University of Leipzig she undertook a residency in the Department of Radiology before becoming consultant and then senior consultant in the Department of Radio-oncology. As well as undertaking fellowships at the Royal Marsden Hospital in London and Surrey and at the Western Infirmary, Glasgow, UK, she trained at the German Cancer Research Institute in Heidelberg. In 1994 she became an assistant professor at the Charité University Hospital in Berlin. She moved in 1999 to the University of Cologne, where she became the professor of Radiation Oncology. Since 2000 she has also been the director of the Clinic of Radiotherapy, Radio-oncology, and Nuclear Medicine at the Vivantes Clinics, Neukölln, Berlin and the professor of Radiation Oncology at the Charité University Medicine Berlin.

Dr Feyer has served as a board member of the MASCC and was its secretary from 2006 to 2008. She is a faculty member of the ESMO, the president of the German Association of Supportive Care in Oncology, Rehabilitation and Social Medicine, the vice president of the Cancer Society of Berlin, and is a member of a number of national and international hematology and oncology societies.

Dr Feyer has authored and coauthored more than 150 articles in national and international journals and books. Her principal areas of clinical interest are quality of life and supportive care in cancer patients, especially minimising side effects of radio and chemotherapy, optimising multimodal treatment strategies in oncology and palliative radio-oncological treatment modalities.

Chapter 1

Introduction

The goal of each antiemetic therapy is to prevent chemotherapy-induced nausea and vomiting (CINV). Few side effects of cancer treatment are more feared by the patient than nausea and vomiting (Figure 1.1) [1,2]. Twenty years ago, these were inevitable adverse events of chemotherapy and forced up to 20% of patients to postpone or refuse potentially curative treatment [3]. Clinical and basic research over the past 25 years has lead to steady improvements in the control of CINV.

Antiemetic agents

For patients with cancer, the development of the serotonin 5-hydroxy-tryptamine-3 (5-HT$_3$) receptor antagonists has been one of the most significant advances in chemotherapy [4]. Corticosteroids show good antiemetic efficacy in the prevention of acute and delayed emesis, especially when combined with other antiemetic agents. However, their role is sometimes underestimated.

Patient perception of the side effects of cancer chemotherapy	
Rank in 1980s	**Rank in 1990s**
1. **Vomiting**	1. Alopecia
2. **Nausea**	2. **Nausea**
3. Alopecia	3. Tiredness
4. Anticipation of treatment	5. Anticipation of treatment
6. Length of treatment in clinic	5. Depression

Figure 1.1 Patient perception of the side effects of cancer chemotherapy. Based on data from Coates et al [1] and Griffin et al [2].

M. Aapro et al., *Prevention of Nausea and Vomiting in Cancer Patients*,
DOI: 10.1007/978-1-907673-58-0_1, © Springer Healthcare 2013

Another group of antiemetics, the neurokinin-1 (NK-1) receptor antagonists, has recently been developed. The first drug in this class, aprepitant, was approved in 2003 [5]. Studies have shown that patients benefit from the use of aprepitant in combination with standard antiemetic therapy, both in the acute and delayed setting of highly and moderately emetogenic chemotherapy.

However, although significant progress has been made with the development of a number of effective and well-tolerated antiemetic treatments, CINV remains an important adverse effect of treatment.

History of antiemetic therapy

The chemotherapy available in the 1950s and 1960s varied greatly in its capacity to induce emesis. Agents such as vinca alkaloids and 5-fluor-uracil were in common usage, and only infrequently caused emesis. In

History of development of chemotherapy and antiemetic therapies for chemotherapy-induced nausea and vomiting	
1950-60	Nitrogen mustard and actinomycin D induce severe emesis
1960	Introduction of phenothiazines → antiemetic effect via dopamin D_2 receptor antagonism
	Borison found that the area postrema is responsible for emesis induced by chemotherapy
1970s	Introduction of cisplatin, no effective antiemetic therapy available
	Case reports of usefulness of cannabinoids
	Metoclopramide found to have antiemetic efficacy
1980s	High-dose metoclopramide improves antiemetic response rates
	Introduction of steroids in prophylaxis
	Studies with GR 38032F (ondansetron)
1990s	Introduction of 5-HT$_3$ receptor antagonists, a milestone in antiemetic therapy
1997	1st Perugia Consensus Conference on antiemetic therapy (MASCC)
2003	Introduction of palonosetron, a second-generation 5-HT$_3$ receptor antagonist
2003	Approval of the first NK-1 receptor antagonist, aprepitant
2004	2nd Perugia Consensus Conference on antiemetic therapy (MASCC/ESMO)
2010	Publication of 3rd Perugia Consensus Conference on antiemetic therapy (MASCC/ESMO)

Figure 1.2 History of development of chemotherapy and antiemetic therapies for chemotherapy-induced nausea and vomiting. 5-HT$_3$, 5-hydroxytryptamine-3; ESMO, European Society of Medical Oncology; MASCC, Multinational Association for Supportive Care in Cancer; NK-1, neurokinin-1.

contrast, nitrogen mustard was known for its association with emesis. There was some awareness of the problem of CINV, but appreciation of its magnitude was not great [6].

A brief historical summary describing the developments of antiemetic treatment is given in Figure 1.2.

References

1 Coates A, Abraham S, Kaye SB, et al. On the receiving end – patient perception of the side-effects of cancer chemotherapy. *Eur J Cancer Clin Oncol*. 1983;19:203-208.
2 Griffin AM, Butow PN, Coates AS, et al. On the receiving end. V: Patient perceptions of the side effects of cancer chemotherapy in 1993. *Ann Oncol*. 1996;7:189-195.
3 Jordan K, Schmoll HJ, Aapro MS. Comparative activity of antiemetic drugs. *Crit Rev Oncol Hematol*. 2007;61:162-175.
4 Aapro MS. Review of experience with ondansetron and granisetron. *Ann Oncol*. 1993; 4(suppl 3):9-14.
5 Hesketh PJ, Grunberg S, Gralla R, et al. The oral neurokinin-1 antagonist aprepitant for the prevention of chemotherapy-induced nausea and vomiting: a multinational, randomised, double-blind, placebo-controlled trial in patients receiving high-dose cisplatin – the Aprepitant Protocol 052 Study Group. *J Clin Oncol*. 2003;21:4112-4119.
6 Gralla RJ. Current issues in the management of nausea and vomiting. *Ann Oncol*. 1993;4(suppl 3):3-7.

Development of this chapter was supported by funding from Helsinn

Chapter 2

Pathophysiology and classification of chemotherapy-induced nausea and vomiting

The pathophysiology of CINV is not entirely understood; however, it is thought to have many contributing pathways. The general mechanisms involved in this highly complex reflex have been elaborated in a number of reviews [1].

Historical background

The central nervous system plays a critical role in the physiology of nausea and vomiting, serving as the primary site that receives and processes a variety of emetic stimuli. The central nervous system also plays a primary role in generating efferent signals, which are sent to a number of organs and tissues in a process that eventually results in vomiting. It was Wang and Borison who first proposed the idea of a vomiting center [2]. However, some of their original observations have not been supported by more recent studies. For example, they showed that vomiting could be induced by stimulation of the dorsolateral medulla in cats, but other investigators have been unable to find a discrete site from which they could consistently elicit vomiting. Moreover, vomiting could still be induced after neuronal cell bodies in the dorsomedial medulla were selectively lesioned. Thus, the simple concept of a vomiting center that could be readily manipulated pharmacologically or surgically has not been upheld [3].

M. Aapro et al., *Prevention of Nausea and Vomiting in Cancer Patients*,
DOI: 10.1007/978-1-907673-58-0_2, © Springer Healthcare 2013

What has been upheld by subsequent research, however, is the original observation that the integrity of the abdominal vagus is essential for emesis [4]. In ferrets, stimulation of mucosal chemoreceptors in the stomach or duodenum by luminal hydrochloride or hypertonic saline results in long latency and sudden increases in vagal efferent discharge associated with the prodrome of vomiting. Thus, signals associated with luminal contents are detected by vagal afferent chemoreceptors in the mucosa and relayed to the hindbrain by a rapid and distinctive fire [5].

Mechanisms of chemotheraphy-induced nausea and vomiting

Three key components involving areas in the hindbrain and the abdominal vagal afferents have been identified (Figure 2.1). Nowadays, it is thought that the existence of an anatomically discrete vomiting centre is unlikely [1]. The locations of neurons that coordinate the bodily functions associated with emesis are spread throughout the medulla, supporting the notion that a central pattern generator coordinates the sequence of

Figure 2.1 Pathways by which chemotherapeutic agents produce an emetic response (opposite). Antineoplastic agents may cause emesis through effects at a number of sites. The mechanism that is best supported by research involves an effect on the upper small intestine (bottom of figure). After the administration of chemotherapy, free radicals are generated, leading to localized exocytotic release of serotonin from the enterochromaffin cells; serotonin then interacts with 5-hydroxytryptamine-3 (5-HT$_3$) receptors on vagal afferent terminals in the wall of the bowel. Vagal afferent fibers project to the dorsal brain stem, primarily to the nucleus tractus solitarius, and, to a lesser extent, the area postrema (AP), the two parts of the brain referred to collectively here as the dorsal vagal complex. Receptors for a number of neurotransmitters with potentially important roles in the emetic response are present in the dorsal vagal complex. These include the neurokinin-1, 5-HT$_3$, and dopamine-2 receptors, which bind to substance P, serotonin and dopamine, respectively. Efferent fibers project from the dorsal vagal complex to the final effecter of the emetic reflex, the central pattern generator, which is an anatomically indistinct area occupying a more ventral location in the brain stem. Receptors for other locally released mediators, such as substance P, cholecystokinin and prostaglandins, are also present on the vagal afferent terminals. However, the extent to which these mediators are involved at this peripheral site is unknown. Antineoplastic agents may also induce emesis through an interaction with the AP within the dorsal vagal complex. The AP is a circumventricular organ located at the caudal end of the floor of the fourth ventricle (see Figure 2.3), which is accessible to blood and cerebrospinal fluid-borne emetic stimuli: it contains the chemoreceptor trigger zone. Other potential sources of efferent input that result in emesis after chemotherapy include a number of structures in the temporal lobe, such as the amygdala. Evidence for this pathway is less well established than for other proposed sites of chemotherapeutic action. 5-HT$_3$, 5-hydroxytryptamine-3; AP, area postrema; NTS, nucleus tractus solitarius. Reproduced with permission from Hesketh [1].

behaviors during emesis. The central pattern generator receives indirect input from both the area postrema (chemoreceptor trigger zone) and the abdominal vagus by means of the nucleus tractus solitarius.

Chemoreceptor trigger zone

The chemoreceptor trigger zone is located in the area postrema at the bottom end of the fourth ventricle. It is a circumventricular organ which basically means that this structure lacks an effective blood–brain barrier and is able to detect emetic agents in both the systemic circulation and

Pathways by which chemotherapeutic agents produce an emetic response

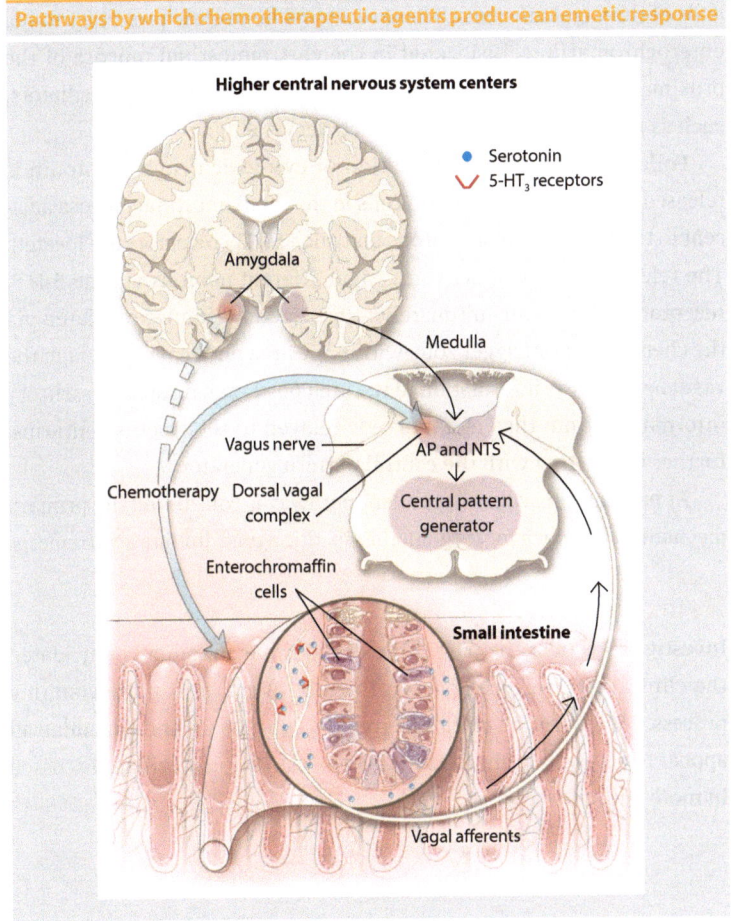

the cerebrospinal fluid. Studies in animal models have demonstrated that opioids and dopaminergic agonists can induce emesis when they bind to this site. The area postrema has afferent and efferent connections with underlying structures, the subnucleus gelatinosus and nucleus tractus solitarius, receiving vagal afferent fibers from the gastrointestinal tract.

Abdominal vagal afferents

The abdominal vagal afferents appear to have the greatest relevance for CINV. A variety of receptors, including 5-hydroxytryptamine-3 (5-HT$_3$), neurokinin-1 (NK-1), and cholecystokinin-1, are located on the terminal ends of the vagal afferents. These receptors lie in close proximity to the enterochromaffin cells located in the gastrointestinal mucosa of the proximal small intestine, which contains a number of local mediators, such as serotonin, substance P, and cholecystokinin.

Following exposure to radiation or cytotoxic drugs, serotonin is released from enterochromaffin cells in the small intestinal mucosa adjacent to the vagal afferent neurons on which 5-HT$_3$ receptors are located. The released serotonin activates vagal afferent neurons via the 5-HT$_3$ receptors, which leads ultimately to an emetic response mediated via the chemoreceptor trigger zone within the area postrema. Although the vagal nerve relays information to the area postrema, most of the sensory information from the vagal nerve is relayed to the tractus solitarius, further interacting with the central pattern generator.

At present, this vagal-dependent pathway is considered the primary mechanism by which most chemotherapeutic agents initiate acute emesis.

Neurotransmitters

Investigations over the past three decades have gradually elucidated the clinical significance of several neurotransmitters in the vomiting process. The neurotransmitters serotonin, substance P and dopamine all appear to play important roles in this process [1,6] and will be discussed in more detail.

Serotonin receptor

Serotonin

Serotonin (or 5-HT) was first isolated in 1948 [7]. As 90% is located in the enterochromaffin cells, it is believed to play the most important role in the process of acute CINV. Following exposure to radiation or cytotoxic drugs, serotonin is released from enterochromaffin cells in the mucosa of the small intestine, which are adjacent to the vagal afferent neurons on which 5-HT$_3$ receptors are located.

5-HT$_3$ receptor

Of the multiple serotonin receptors identified to date, the 5-HT$_3$ receptor appears to be most important in the acute phase of CINV although a role in the delayed phase cannot be totally ruled out. The 5-HT$_3$ receptor is the only monoamine neurotransmitter receptor that functions as a ligand-operated ion channel (Figure 2.2). It has been identified only in neurons, in the central and peripheral autonomic, sensory, and enteric systems. The highest densities of 5-HT$_3$ receptors in the brain are located in the area postrema, nucleus tractus solitarius, and dorsal vagal motor nucleus,

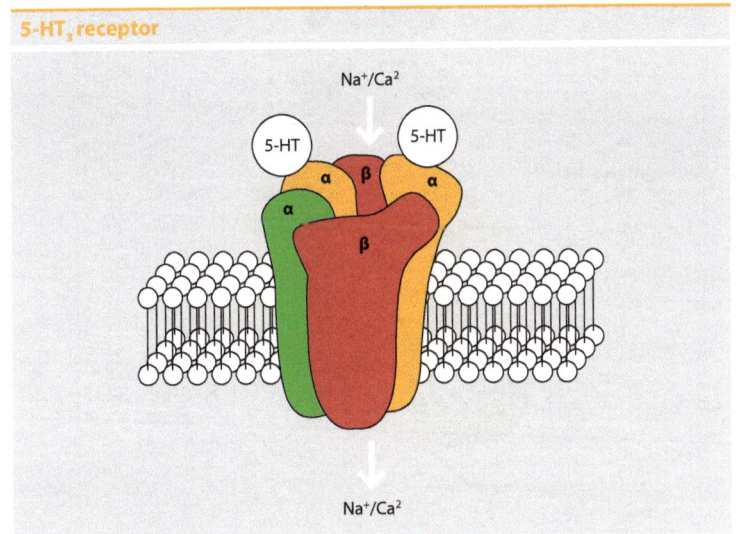

Figure 2.2 5-HT$_3$ receptor. 5-HT, 5-hydroxytryptamine; 5-HT$_3$, 5-Hydroxytryptamine-3.

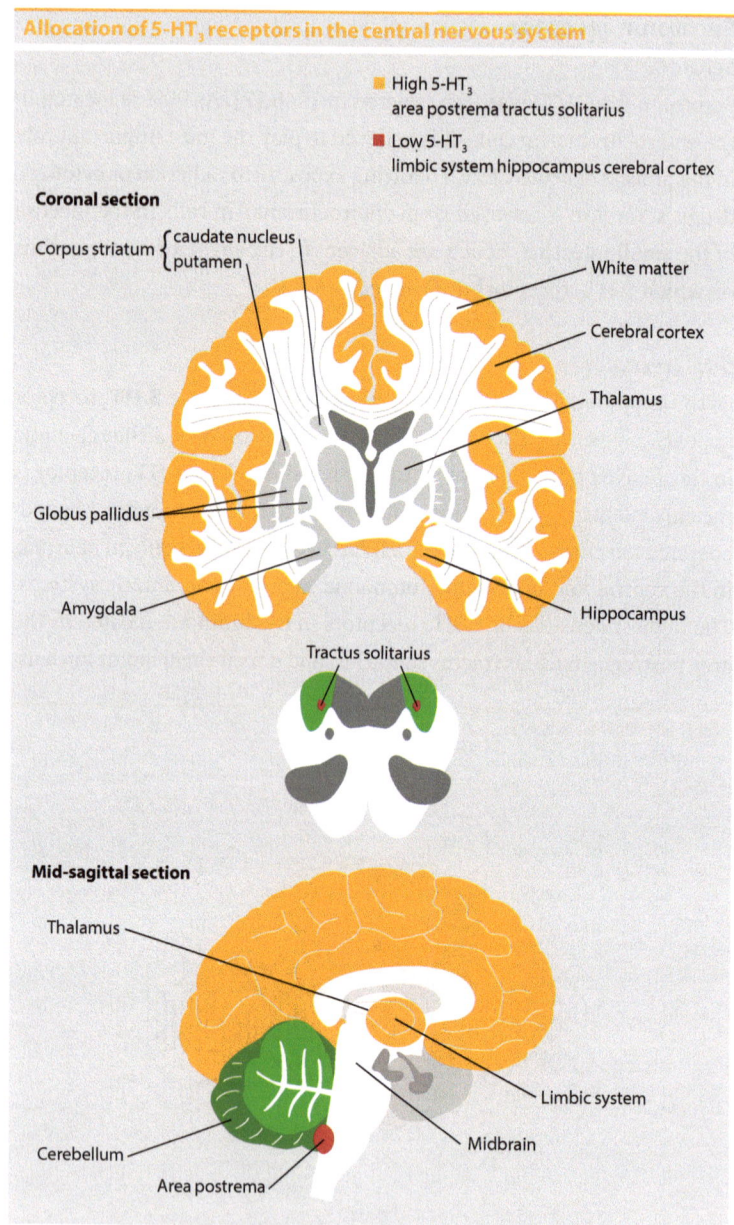

Figure 2.3 Allocation of 5-HT₃ receptors in the central nervous system. $5\text{-}HT_3$, 5-hydroxytryptamine-3 receptor. Based on data from Miller et al [8], Moulignier [9], and Peroutka et al [10].

as depicted in Figure 2.3. They mediate a rapid depolarizing response associated with an increase in membrane conductance following the opening of cation-selective channels; the influx of sodium and calcium contribute importantly to the response. The response to serotonin is usually described as a cooperative effect, in which the occupation of one receptor subunit enhances the binding of other agonist molecules. The 5-HT$_3$ receptor has probably evolved to mediate rapid synaptic events. However, it should be noted that in all 5-HT$_3$ systems examined, repeated challenge to serotonin is met by desensitization and a rapid decline in the amplitude of depolarization.

The hypothesis that 5-HT$_3$ receptor antagonists (RAs) might be useful as antiemetics was based on the results of several studies, including the findings that metoclopramide is a weak 5-HT$_3$-RAs and that high-dose metoclopramide is effective against cisplatin-induced emesis [11]. These findings led to the development of selective serotonin RAs and the publication of the first clinical study of a 5-HT$_3$-RA in 1987 [12].

Substance P and neurokinin-1 receptor

Substance P was first discovered in 1931, yet its molecular target was not identified until several decades later [13]. Early research to elucidate the role of this peptide focused on its behavioral and physiological effects in the central and peripheral nervous system. Substance P, the natural ligand of the NK-1 receptor, has been shown to be involved in the transmission of unpleasant stimuli, such as pain, mood disorders, anxiety, stress, and nausea and vomiting. Substance P is a neuropeptide that acts as a neurotransmitter or neuromodulator within both the central and peripheral nervous system by preferentially binding to the NK-1 receptor (Figure 2.4). During the past two decades, multiple studies have suggested that substance P may also be a relevant neurotransmitter in CINV [14]. In early studies it was shown that administration of substance P to dogs could induce emesis [15]. In further studies, several selective NK-1 receptor antagonists in animal models revealed substantial antiemetic efficacy across a broad spectrum of emetic stimuli.

Neurokinin-1 receptor

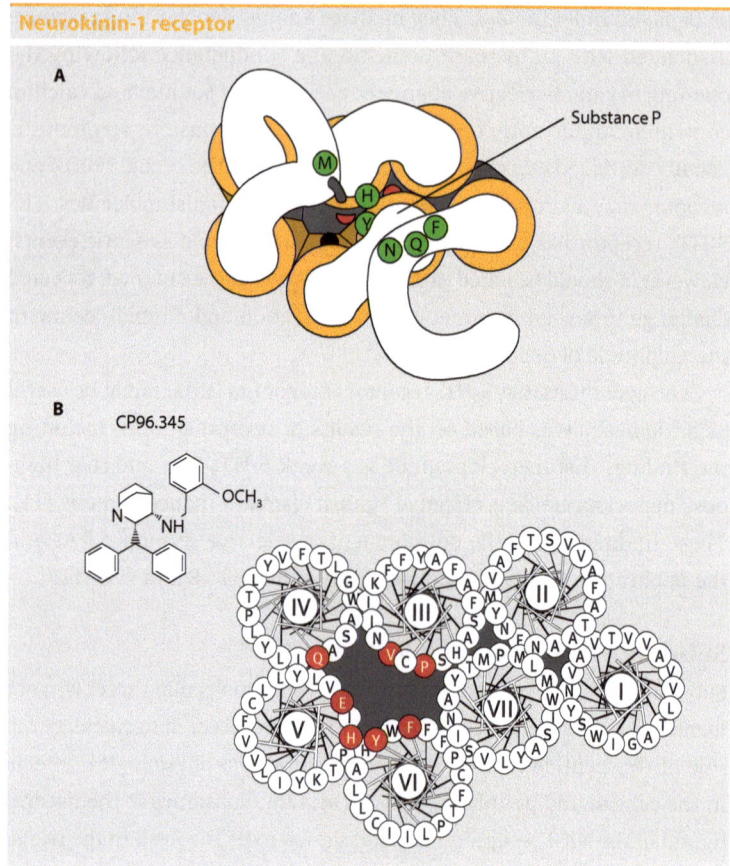

Figure 2.4 Neurokinin-1 receptor. A, The interaction sides for substance P are shown as green circles; B, The seven transmembrane segments are shown as helical wheels (I to VII), and the interaction points for the prototype nonpeptide antagonist CP-96,345 are shown by red circles. Reproduced with permission from Hokfelt et al [13].

Dopamine

Dopamine interacts with dopamine D_1 and D_2 receptors. The dopamine D_2 receptor, located in the chemoreceptor trigger zone, is in part responsible for chemotherapy-induced emesis. In early antiemetic trials in the 1960s, attention was mostly paid to agents that block dopamine receptors. Today, it is recognized that the antiemetic effect of high-dose metoclopramide is probably due to 5-HT$_3$ receptor antagonism [16]. Certain adverse events associated with dopamine D_2-receptor antagonism include hyperprolactinemia and extrapyramidal symptoms (eg, akinesia, acute dystonic reactions) [17].

Classification of nausea and vomiting

CINV may be classified into three categories (Figures 2.5 and 2.6):

- **acute onset,** occurring within 24 hours of initial administration of chemotherapy;
- **delayed onset,** occurring 24 hours to several days after initial treatment; and
- **anticipatory nausea and vomiting,** observed in patients whose emetic episodes are triggered by taste, odor, sight, thoughts, or anxiety secondary to a history of poor response to antiemetic agents [19,20].

Three categories of chemotherapy-induced nausea and vomiting
Acute nausea and vomiting
Within the first 24 hours after chemotherapy
Mainly by serotonin release from the enterochromaffin cells
Delayed nausea and vomiting
After 24 hours to 5 days after chemotherapy
Various mechanisms: mainly substance P mediated, disruption of the blood–brain barrier, disruption of the gastrointestinal motility, adrenal hormones (Roila et al [19])
Anticipatory nausea and vomiting
Occurrence is possible after 1 cycle of chemotherapy (Aapro et al [20])
Involves an element of classic conditioning

Figure 2.5 Three categories of chemotherapy-induced nausea and vomiting. Adapted from Jordan et al [18].

Classification of chemotherapy-induced nausea and vomiting

Figure 2.6 Classification of chemotherapy-induced nausea and vomiting.

References

1   Hesketh PJ. Chemotherapy-induced nausea and vomiting. *N Engl J Med*. 2008;358:2482-2494.

2   Wang SC, Borison HL. The vomiting center; a critical experimental analysis. *Arch Neurol Psychiatry*. 1950;63:928-941.

3   Andrews PL, Horn CC. Signals for nausea and emesis: Implications for models of upper gastrointestinal diseases. *Auton Neurosci*. 2006;125:100-115.

4   Miller FR . On gastric sensation. *J Physiol*. 1910;41:409-415.

5   Hornby PJ. Central neurocircuitry associated with emesis. *Am J Med*. 2001;111(suppl 8A):106S-112S.

6   Gralla RJ. Current issues in the management of nausea and vomiting. *Ann Oncol*. 1993;4(suppl 3):3-7.

7   Rapport MM, Green AA, Page IH. Crystalline serotonin. *Science*. 1948;108:329-330.

8   Miller AD, Nonaka S, Jakus J. Brain areas essential or non-essential for emesis. *Brain Res*. 1994;647:255-264.

9   Moulignier A. [Central serotonin receptors. Principal fundamental and functional aspects. Therapeutic applications]. *Rev Neurol (Paris)*. 1994;150:3-15.

10 Peroutka SJ, Snyder SH. Two distinct serotonin receptors: regional variations in receptor binding in mammalian brain. *Brain Res*. 1981;208:339-347.

11 Gralla RJ, Itri LM, Pisko SE, et al. Antiemetic efficacy of high-dose metoclopramide: randomized trials with placebo and prochlorperazine in patients with chemotherapy-induced nausea and vomiting. *N Engl J Med*. 1981;305:905-909.

12 Leibundgut U, Lancranjan I. First results with ICS 205-930 (5-HT 3 receptor antagonist) in prevention of chemotherapy-induced emesis. *Lancet*. 1987;1:1198.

13 Hokfelt T, Pernow B, Wahren J. Substance P: a pioneer amongst neuropeptides. *J Intern Med*. 2001;249:27-40.

14 Kris MG, Radford JE, Pizzo BA, et al. Use of an NK1 receptor antagonist to prevent delayed emesis after cisplatin. *J Natl Cancer Inst*. 1997;89:817-818.

15 Carpenter DO, Briggs DB, Strominger N. Responses of neurons of canine area postrema to neurotransmitters and peptides. *Cell Mol Neurobiol*. 1983;3:113-126.

16 Herrstedt J, Dombernowsky P. Anti-emetic therapy in cancer chemotherapy: current status. *Basic Clin Pharmacol Toxicol*. 2007;101:143-150.

17 Tonini M, Cipollina L, Poluzzi E, et al. Review article: clinical implications of enteric and central D2 receptor blockade by antidopaminergic gastrointestinal prokinetics. *Aliment Pharmacol Ther*. 2004;19:379-390.

18 Jordan K, Schmoll HJ, Aapro MS. Comparative activity of antiemetic drugs. *Crit Rev Oncol Hematol*. 2007;61:162-175.

19 Roila F, Donati D, Tamberi S, Margutti G. Delayed emesis: incidence, pattern, prognostic factors and optimal treatment. *Support Care Cancer*. 2002;10:88-95.

20 Aapro MS, Molassiotis A, Olver I. Anticipatory nausea and vomiting. *Support Care Cancer*. 2005;13:117-121.

Development of this chapter was supported by funding from Helsinn

Risk factors associated with nausea and vomiting after chemotherapy

The severity and clinical presentation of CINV depend on several factors. The emetogenic potential of the chemotherapeutic agents used is the main risk factor for the degree of CINV. Individual patient characteristics, which may differ substantially from one patient to another, must also be taken into consideration.

Emetogenic potential of chemotherapy

It is thought that this is the most important risk factor for the occurrence of CINV. The emetogenic potential of chemotherapeutic agents is classified into four emetic risk groups: high, moderate, low and minimal [1–3], as shown in Figure 3.1.

The emetogenic potential of an antineoplastic therapy varies with the specific drug used (Figures 3.2. and 3.3), ranging from cisplatin, which results in severe vomiting in almost all patients, to vinca alkaloids,

Classification of emetogenic potential		
Emesis-risk	**Acute emesis**	**Delayed emesis**
High (>90%)	++	++
Moderate (30–90%)	++	+
Low (10–30%)	+	–
Minimal (<10%)	–	–

Figure 3.1 Classification of emetogenic potential. + high emesis risk; – minimal emesis-risk. Based on data from Hesketh et al [2] and Koeller et al [4].

M. Aapro et al., *Prevention of Nausea and Vomiting in Cancer Patients*, DOI: 10.1007/978-1-907673-58-0_3, © Springer Healthcare 2013

Emetogenic risk of intravenous chemotherapeutic agents

High (emesis risk >90% without antiemetics)

Actinomycin D	Lomustine
Carmustine	Mechlorethamine
Cisplatin	Pentostatin
Cyclophosphamide (>1500 mg/m^2)	Streptozotocin
Dacarbazine	

Moderate (emesis risk 30–90% without antiemetics)

Alemtuzumab	Epirubicin
Altretamine	Idarubicin
Azacitidine	Ifosfamide
Bendamustine	Irinotecan
Clofarabine	Melphalan IV
Carboplatin	Mitoxantrone (>12 mg/m^2)
Cyclophosphamide (<1500 mg/m^2)	Oxaliplatin
Cytarabine (>1 g/m^2)	Temozolomide
Daunorubicin	Treosulphan
Doxorubicin	Trabectedin

Low (emesis risk 10–30% without antiemetics)

Asparaginase	Methotrexate (>100 mg/m^2)
Bortezomib	Mitoxantrone (<12 mg/m^2)
Catumaxomab	Paclitaxel
Cetuximab	Panitumumab
Cytarabine (<1 g/m^2)	Pegasparaginase
Docetaxel	Pemetrexed
Doxorubicin liposomal	Teniposide
Etoposide IV	Thiotepa
5-Fluorouracil	Topotecan
Gemcitabine	Trastuzumab
Ixabepilone	

Minimal (emesis risk <10% without antiemetics)

Bleomycin	Hydroxyurea
Bevacizumab	α-, β-, γ- Interferon
Busulphan	Mercaptopurine
Chlorambucil	Methotrexate (<100 mg/m^2)
Cladribine	Thioguanine
Cytarabine (<100 mg/m^2)	Vinblastine
Fludarabin	Vincristine
Hormones	Vinorelbine

Figure 3.2 Emetogenic risk of intravenous chemotherapeutic agents. Based on data from Jordan et al [5], Kris et al [3], NCCN [6] and Roila et al [7,8].

Emetogenic risk of oral chemotherapeutic agents	
High (emesis risk >90% without antiemetics)	
Hexamethylmelamine	Procarbazine
Moderate (emesis risk 30–90% without antiemetics)	
Cyclophosphamide	Temozolomide
Imatinib	Vinorelbine
Low (emesis risk 10–30% without antiemetics)	
Capecitabine	Lapatinib
Etoposide	Lenalidomide
Everolimus	Sunitinib
Fludarabine	Thalidomide
Minimal (emesis risk <10% without antiemetics)	
Chlorambucil	Melphalan
Erlotinib	Methotrexate
Gefitinib	Sorafenib
Hydroxyurea	6-Thioguanine

Figure 3.3 Emetogenic risk of oral chemotherapeutic agents. Based on data from Jordan et al [5], NCCN [6], and Roila et al [7,8].

with only minimal inducible emesis. The chemotherapeutic agents can cause different intensities of emesis, depending on the way the drugs are administered. The same drug, when given as a bolus injection, can cause more severe emesis than a continuous infusion because the peak levels of drug concentration *in vivo* are higher with short time application.

Patient risk factors
Previous experience of poorly controlled emesis
If patients have previous experience of poorly controlled emesis they are more likely to develop post-chemotherapy nausea and vomiting in response to a new treatment. Here it is not only the occurrence of emesis in the past that is important, but also the degree of the side effects experienced. If emetic control was sufficient during previous chemotherapy, the percentage of patients who do not experience emesis in subsequent chemotherapy courses is larger than it is for patients who had insufficient previous antiemetic treatment [9].

Sex and age

Sex is probably also one of the most important individual prognostic factors in predicting CINV: female gender predisposes to CINV. Age also appears to be an important risk factor that influences nausea and vomiting after chemotherapy. Younger patients (ie, <50 years) experience more severe nausea and vomiting after chemotherapy than older patients (>65 years).

Alcohol intake

Alcohol intake is another factor that can influence the level of CINV. Studies have indicated that a history of chronic heavy alcohol abuse (>100 g/day) may be associated with better control of CINV [9,10]. It has been assumed that chronic alcohol exposure results in a decreased sensitivity of the chemoreceptor trigger zone, but knowledge of this area is still incomplete. However, it is of note that a low alcohol intake on a regular basis is associated with a lower control of CINV.

History of motion sickness

A history of motion sickness is also a contributing factor for the development of CINV. It has been found that patients susceptible to motion sickness report both a greater frequency of nausea following chemotherapy and a greater severity and longer duration of each episode of post-treatment emesis.

Other factors

Further patient characteristics that contribute to risk for CINV are given in Figure 3.4.

Summary

The characteristics of affected patients suggest a large group of factors that can, each by itself or in combination, modulate the occurrence of nausea and vomiting after chemotherapy.

Patient characteristics influencing the occurrence of chemotherapy-induced nausea and vomiting

Risk factor	Raised (↑) or decreased risk (↓)
Experience of nausea and or vomiting during previous chemotherapy	↑
Age <50 years	↑
Female gender	↑
Anxiety	↑
Pretreatment nausea	↑
Chemotherapy as an inpatient	↓
Chemotherapy as an outpatient	↑
Severe alcohol consumption	↓
Low intake of alcohol	↑
Impaired quality of life	↑
History of motion sickness	↑
Pain	↑
Vomiting during pregnancy	↑
Fatigue	↑

Figure 3.4 Patient characteristics influencing the occurrence of chemotherapy-induced nausea and vomiting. Based on data from Hesketh [11], Jordan et al [12], and Morrow et al [13].

References

1 Grunberg SM, Osoba D, Hesketh PJ, et al. Evaluation of new antiemetic agents and definition of antineoplastic agent emetogenicity – an update. *Support Care Cancer*. 2005; 13: 80-84.
2 Hesketh PJ, Kris MG, Grunberg SM, et al. Proposal for classifying the acute emetogenicity of cancer chemotherapy. *J Clin Oncol*. 1997; 15: 103-109.
3 Kris MG, Hesketh PJ, Somerfield MR, et al. American Society of Clinical Oncology guideline for antiemetics in oncology: update 2006. *J Clin Oncol*. 2006; 24: 2932-2947.
4 Koeller JM, Aapro MS, Gralla RJ, et al. Antiemetic guidelines: creating a more practical treatment approach. *Support Care Cancer*. 2002; 10: 519-522.
5 Jordan K, Sippel C, Schmoll HJ. Guidelines for antiemetic treatment of chemotherapy-induced nausea and vomiting: past, present, and future recommendations. *Oncologist*. 2007; 12:1143-1150.
6 National Comprehensive Cancer Network. *Antiemesis, Clinical Practice Guidelines in Oncology*. Fort Washington, PA: National Comprehensive Cancer Network; 2010.
7 Roila F, Hesketh PJ, Herrstedt J. Prevention of chemotherapy- and radiotherapy-induced emesis: results of the 2004 Perugia International Antiemetic Consensus Conference. *Ann Oncol*. 2006;17:20-28.
8 Roila F, Herrstedt J, Aapro M, et al. Guideline update for MASCC and ESMO in the prevention of chemotherapy- and radiotherapy-induced nausea and vomiting: results of the Perugia consensus conference *Ann Oncol*. 2010:21(suppl 5):v232–v243.
9 Gralla RJ, Osoba D, Kris MG, et al. Recommendations for the use of antiemetics: evidence-based, clinical practice guidelines. American Society of Clinical Oncology. *J Clin Oncol*. 1999; 17: 2971-2974.

10 Roila F, Tonato M, Cognetti F, et al. Prevention of cisplatin-induced emesis: a double-blind multicenter randomised crossover study comparing ondansetron and ondansetron plus dexamethasone. *J Clin Oncol*. 1991;9:675-678.

11 Hesketh PJ. Chemotherapy-induced nausea and vomiting. *N Engl J Med*. 2008;358:2482-2494.

12 Jordan K, Grothey A, Pelz T, et al. Impact of quality of life parameters and coping strategies on postchemotherapy nausea and vomiting (PCNV). *Eur J Cancer Care*. 2009;19:603–609.

13 Morrow GR, Roscoe JA, Hickok JT, et al. Nausea and emesis: evidence for a biobehavioral perspective. *Support Care Cancer*. 2002;10:96-105.

Development of this chapter was supported by funding from Helsinn

Risk factors associated with nausea and vomiting after radiotherapy

One of the main stumbling blocks in devising effective treatment of radiotherapy-induced nausea and vomiting (RINV) has been a lack of consensus on the emetic potential of different radiotherapy techniques and doses. The literature that is available suggests that extent of irradiation is one of the major determinants of risk for RINV. The Multinational Association of Supportive Care in Cancer/European Society of Medical Oncology (MASCC/ESMO) guidelines from 2009 and the guidelines from the American Society of Clinical Oncology (ASCO) from 2006 divided the risk of emesis due to radiotherapy into four categories based upon the radiation field [1,2], as described below.

Classification of radiotherapy-induced nausea and vomiting

- High (risk of emesis >90%): total body irradiation (TBI).
- Moderate (risk of emesis 60–90%): upper abdominal irradiation, half body irradiation (HBI) and upper body irradiation (UBI).
- Low (risk of emesis 30–60%): cranium (all), craniospinal, head and neck, lower thorax region, pelvis.
- Minimal (risk of emesis <30%): other sites, including breast and extremities.

In view of the results from two newer studies, in the new guidelines head and neck radiation and brain radiation have been reclassified as belonging to the low emetogenic risk group, in contrast to their status

M. Aapro et al., *Prevention of Nausea and Vomiting in Cancer Patients*, 21
DOI: 10.1007/978-1-907673-58-0_4, © Springer Healthcare 2013

in the ASCO guidelines from 2006 [3,4]. In addition to the irradiated area, concomitant chemotherapy, field size, and dose per fraction are also important risk factors.

References

1 Feyer P, Maranzano M, Molassiotis A, et al. Radiotherapy-induced nausea and vomiting (RINV): MASCC/ESMO Guideline for Antiemetics in Radiotherapy: update 2009. *Support Care Cancer.* 2011(suppl 1):S5-S14.
2 Kris MG, Hesketh PJ, Somerfield MR, et al. American Society of Clinical Oncology guideline for antiemetics in oncology: update 2006. *J Clin Oncol.* 2006;24:2932-47.
3 Enblom A, Bergius Axelsson B, Steineck G, et al. One third of patients with radiotherapy-induced nausea consider their antiemetic treatment insufficient. *Support Care Cancer.* 2009;17:23-32.
4 Maranzano E, De Angelis V, Pergolizzi S, et al. Radiation-induced emesis (RIE): results of the second observational multicenter Italian trial. *Radiother Oncol.* 2010;1:36-41.

Development of this chapter was supported by funding from Helsinn

Chapter 5

Antiemetic drugs

With modern antiemetics, vomiting can be completely prevented in up to 70–80% of patients [1–3]. Combination antiemetic regimens have become the standard of care for the control of chemotherapy-induced nausea and vomiting (CINV) [4].

Several classes of antiemetic drugs are available that antagonize the neurotransmitter receptors responsible for CINV. The antiemetic drugs are classified according to their primary action (Figure 5.1) and have different efficacy in the acute and delayed phase of emesis.

Serotonin receptor antagonists

The 5-hydroxytryptamine-3 receptor antagonists (5-HT$_3$-RAs) are without doubt the most effective antiemetics in the prophylaxis of acute CINV. The wide experience acquired with these drugs in daily clinical practice since the early 1990s has confirmed their remarkable safety profile [4]. The 5-HT$_3$-RAs form the cornerstone of therapy for the control of acute emesis in the context of chemotherapy agents that have moderate to high emetogenic potential. Furthermore, additional studies on these agents suggest that particular 5-HT$_3$-RAs have value in the treatment of delayed emesis associated with chemotherapy as well.

Five 5-HT$_3$-RAs are available: dolasetron, granisetron, ondansetron, palonosetron, and tropisetron. In a meta-analysis comparing the four older 5-HT$_3$-RAs (dolasetron, granisetron, ondansetron, and tropisetron), the 5-HT$_3$-RAs were equally effective, though there was an advantage

M. Aapro et al., *Prevention of Nausea and Vomiting in Cancer Patients*, 23
DOI: 10.1007/978-1-907673-58-0_5, © Springer Healthcare 2013

Antiemetics: site of action and examples

Site of action	Class/drug	Examples
5-HT$_3$ receptor	5-HT$_3$ receptor antagonist	Ondansetron
		Granisetron
		Palonosetron
		Tropisetron
		Dolasetron
Multiple	Steroids	Dexamethasone
		Methylprednisolone
Neurokinin-1 receptor	Neurokinin-1 receptor antagonist	Aprepitant
		Fosaprepitant
Dopamine-D$_2$ receptor	Substituted benzamides	Metoclopramide
		Alizapride
GABA-Chloride channel receptor complex	Benzodiazepines	Lorazepam
		Diazepam
Dopamine-D$_2$ receptor	Neuroleptics	Promethazine
		Haloperidol
Multiple	Atypical neuroleptics	Olanzapine
Cannabinoid receptor	Cannabinoids	Dronabinol
		Nabilone
Muscarinic cholinergic receptor	Antihistamines	Dimenhydrinate

Figure 5.1 Antiemetics: site of action and examples. 5-HT$_3$, 5-hydroxytryptamine-3; GABA, gamma-aminobutyric acid.

for granisetron when compared directly with tropisetron [5–7]. The guideline-based dose recommendations are shown in Figure 5.2.

Palonosetron differs from the other four 5-HT$_3$-RAs in having a higher receptor binding affinity, longer half-life (see product leaflets for reference), and a different mechanism of action, exhibiting allosteric binding and positive cooperativity to the 5-HT$_3$ receptor, instead of simple bimolecular binding, and triggering receptor internalisation and prolonged inhibition of receptor function [8] (Figure 5.3). Recent findings have also shown that palonosetron uniquely inhibits crosstalk between the 5-HT$_3$ and neurokinin-1 (NK-1) receptor pathways in a dose- and time-dependent fashion [9]. These different features may lead to better efficacy in the delayed phase of CINV [10,11]. Phase III trials in the setting of moderately emetogenic chemotherapy have suggested higher efficacy compared with first generation 5-HT$_3$-RAs, dolasetron and ondansetron [15,16]. In view of

Dose of antiemetics

5-HT₃ receptor antagonist	Route	Recommended dose
Ondansetron	PO	24 mg (high) 16 mg* (moderate)
	IV	8 mg (0.15 mg/kg)
Granisetron	PO	2 mg
	IV	1 mg (0.01 mg/kg)
Tropisetron	PO	5 mg
	IV	5 mg
Dolasetron	PO	100 mg
Palonosetron	IV	0.25 mg
	PO	0.5 mg
Steroids		
Dexamethasone	PO/IV	12 mg (high emetogenic with aprepitant) 20 mg w/o aprepitant
		8 mg (moderate emetogenic), 8 mg (high/moderate) days 2, 3
NK-1 receptor antagonist		
Aprepitant	PO	125 mg day 1, 80 mg days 2 + 3
Fosaprepitant		115 mg day 1 (IV), 80 mg days 2 + 3 (orally) or
		150 mg only on 1 day (IV)

Figure 5.2 Dose of antiemetics. *8 mg twice daily is recommended. Based on data from Jordan et al [2], Kris et al [12], and Roila et al [13,14].

Pharmacokinetic parameters of 5-HT₃ receptor antagonists

	Ondansetron	Granisetron	Tropisetron	Dolasetron	Palonosetron
Half-life (h)	4.0	9.0	8.0	7.5	40
Receptor binding constant, pK_i	8.1	8.4	8.8	7.6	10.5

Figure 5.3 Pharmacokinetic parameters of 5-HT₃ receptor antagonists. See product leaflets for reference.

these results, and because it has been shown and generally agreed that no major differences in terms of efficacy exist between the four older 5-HT₃ receptor antagonists mentioned above [5–7,14], the updated MASCC 2009 guidelines recommend palonosetron as the preferred agent in patients receiving non-anthracycline/cyclophosphamide moderate emetogenic chemotherapy, as well as in those receiving anthracycline/cyclophospha-mide therapy if a NK-1-RA is unavailable [14].

In the latest study in Japan [17], the efficacy of a 0.75 mg dose of palonosetron (approved dose in Japan) plus dexamethasone versus a 40 µg/kg dose of granisetron plus dexamethasone was evaluated in patients receiving cisplatin-based or anthracycline plus cyclophosphamide-based regimens. In this phase III study, prevention of CINV with palonosetron and granisetron was comparable at the end of day 1. However, palonosetron demonstrated statistically superior CINV prevention in the delayed phase; the complete response rate was 56.8% with palonosetron/dexamethasone versus 44.5% with granisetron/dexamethasone ($P < 0.0001$) [17].

Dose recommendation

When administering 5-HT$_3$-RAs, several points should be taken into consideration [18–20]:

- The lowest fully effective dose for each agent should be used (Figure 5.2); because receptors become saturated, higher doses do not enhance any aspect of activity.
- Oral and intravenous routes are equally effective although the injection form of dolasetron is no longer used to prevent CINV (see below).
- No schedule is better than a single dose given before chemotherapy.

Side effects

The adverse effects of 5-HT$_3$-RAs are generally mild, with headache, constipation, diarrhea and asthenia mainly described [21]. Small, transient, reversible changes in electrocardiographic parameters have been shown to occur with some available 5-HT$_3$-RAs (please consult the Prescribing Information/Summary of Product Characteristics of each specific product to find possible differences in precaution warnings, especially for any patient having a risk of QTc prolongation). Since 2010, following an FDA warning, the injection form of dolasetron is no longer used to prevent CINV in pediatric and adult patients (http://www.fda.gov/drugs/drugsafety/ucm237081.htm.). This was in response to data showing that dolasetron injection can increase the risk of developing an abnormal heart rhythm (torsade de pointes), which in some cases can be fatal. Dolasetron tablets may still be used to prevent CINV because the risk of developing an abnormal heart rhythm with the oral form of this drug is less than that seen with the injection form.

Steroids

Steroids are an integral part of antiemetic therapy for acute and delayed CINV, although they are not approved as antiemetics [22]. When used in combination with other antiemetics, corticosteroids exert a booster effect, raising the emetic threshold.

Dexamethasone is the most frequently used corticosteroid, although no study reports the superiority of one corticosteroid over another in terms of efficacy [19]. Besides the recently introduced NK-1-RAs, dexamethasone is one of the most important drugs in preventing delayed CINV [23].

Dose recommendation

For prevention of acute CINV, the dexamethasone dose of choice should be 20 mg (12 mg when coadministered with aprepitant) in highly emetogenic chemotherapy (HEC) and a single dose of 8 mg dexamethasone in moderately emetogenic chemotherapy (MEC) (Figure 5.2) [24,25] has been recommended by the ESMO/MASCC and ASCO guidelines [12,14]. For use of dexamethasone in delayed emesis, the suggested dose is 8 mg PO/IV.

Side effects

Steroids are considered to be safe antiemetics. Side effects are usually dependent on dose and duration of therapy. However, in a study of patients receiving dexamethasone for the prophylaxis of delayed CINV, patients reported moderate to severe problems with insomnia (45%), indigestion/epigastric discomfort (27%), agitation (27%), increased appetite (19%), weight gain (16%), and acne (15%) in the week following chemotherapy [26]. In a recently published study of palonosetron plus dexamethasone on day 1 with or without dexamethasone on days 2 and 3, 8.7% of patients receiving dexamethasone for up to 3 days had insomnia, vs. 2.6% of those receiving dexamethasone for only 1 day [27]. Concerns that steroids may interfere with the antitumor effects of chemotherapy through immunosuppressive mechanisms have not been confirmed in clinical trials [28]. Dexamethasone-sparing regimens on days 2 and 3, in combination with palonosetron, have recently been studied and have shown promising results [27].

Neurokinin-1 receptor antagonists

Aprepitant is the first representative of this new group and blocks the NK-1 receptor in the brainstem (central pattern generator) and gastrointestinal tract [1]. Aprepitant is currently the only agent available in this class, although a novel NK-1-RA, namely casopitant, has shown clinical promise in phase III trials of patients receiving MEC and HEC.

Aprepitant

Regimens containing aprepitant plus a $5\text{-}HT_3$-RA and a corticosteroid have been shown to significantly reduce acute and delayed emesis in patients receiving HEC [1,2,29] and MEC, compared with regimens containing a $5\text{-}HT_3$-RA plus dexamethasone only [30,31]. The standard use of triple therapy including aprepitant (or fosaprepitant), a $5\text{-}HT_3$ receptor antagonist and dexamethasone is currently recommended in HEC and anthracycline-based chemotherapy [14].

Dose recommendation

A randomized study established the most favorable risk profile of aprepitant at doses of 125 mg PO on day 1 and 80 mg PO on days 2 and 3 (Figure 5.2) [32].

Fosaprepitant

A parenteral formulation of aprepitant (fosaprepitant, a water-soluble pro-drug of aprepitant) is now available. The dose is 115 mg IV 30 minutes prior to chemotherapy on day 1, followed by 80 mg of aprepitant orally on days 2 and 3. The finding that a single dose of fosaprepitant (150 mg IV) is equally effective as the 3-day oral aprepitant regimen, as reported at ASCO 2010, supports this more convenient mode of administration of the NK-1-RA [33].

Side effects

In general, the incidence of adverse events reported with aprepitant plus 5-HT$_3$-RA and dexamethasone is similar to that with 5-HT$_3$-RA plus dexamethasone alone: headache, 8% versus 10%; anorexia, 12% versus 11%; asthenia/fatigue, 20% versus 17%; diarrhea, 11% versus 12%; hiccups, 12% versus 9% [34].

Interactions

Aprepitant is metabolized by cytochrome P450 (CYP) 3A4. It is a moderate inhibitor and an inducer of CYP3A4 [35]. Aprepitant has been shown to cause a two-fold increase in the area under the plasma concentration curve of dexamethasone, which is a sensitive substrate of CYP3A4. Consequently, dexamethasone doses should be decreased by approximately 50% when used in combination with aprepitant [35–38]. Potential interactions with cytotoxic drugs metabolized by CYP3A4 have been intensively studied: aprepitant has no clinically significant effect on either the pharmacokinetics or toxicity of standard doses of docetaxel in cancer patients [39], and the metabolism of cyclophosphamide is not significantly reduced in the presence of aprepitant [40]. A recent review has confirmed that there is no proven clinically significant interaction with intravenous cytotoxic agents, but caution with oral agents is still recommended [23].

Casopitant

The investigational drug casopitant is a potent, selective, competitive NK-1-RA, under development at the time of writing. However, the manufacturer has discontinued regulatory filing on a worldwide basis for casopitant because significant further safety data would be required to support registration.

Dopamine receptor antagonists

Prior to the introduction of 5-HT$_3$-RAs, dopamine receptor antagonists formed the basis of antiemetic therapy [6]. These agents can be subdivided into phenothiazines, butyrophenones, and substituted benzamides [6,41]. One of the most frequently used benzamides is metoclopramide. Before the 5-HT$_3$-RAs became established in CINV prophylaxis, metoclopramide, usually at high doses and in combination with a corticosteroid, played a primary role in the management of acute CINV. However, in patients receiving cisplatin-based chemotherapy, the effects of conventional doses of metoclopramide are not significantly different from placebo. Consequently, current guidelines do not recommend metoclopramide for prevention of acute CINV.

Although not effective in the acute phase, metoclopramide in combination with corticosteroids has proven efficacy in the prevention of delayed CINV [42,43]. Indeed, it has been demonstrated that metoclopramide-containing regimens are more effective than corticosteroid monotherapy. In the study by the Italian Group for Antiemetic Research, the combination of metoclopramide plus corticosteroid was shown to be as effective as 5-HT$_3$-RA plus corticosteroid in the delayed phase (complete response: 60% vs 62%) [44]. Consequently, metoclopramide was recommended for the prevention of delayed CINV by the first MASCC and former ASCO antiemetic guidelines [19]. However, in the updated MASCC and ASCO guidelines, metoclopramide is no longer recommended for use in the prevention of delayed CINV [12,14] due to the availability of more effective antiemetic drugs. The current guidelines recommend that metoclopramide should be reserved for patients intolerant of or refractory to 5-HT$_3$-RAs, dexamethasone and aprepitant [12,14].

Olanzapine

Olanzapine, an atypical antipsychotic drug, has potential antiemetic properties due to its ability to antagonize several neurotransmitters involved in the CINV pathways. Adverse effects reported are typical of those seen with other antipsychotics and include sleepiness, dizziness, weight gain, and dry mouth but usually no extrapyramidal side effects [41].

In a phase II study, olanzapine demonstrated effective prevention of both acute and delayed CINV in patients receiving HEC or MEC [45]. Consequently, olanzapine is cited in the updated guidelines as a potential treatment option for refractory and breakthrough emesis [14,46]. Further studies are currently underway to further elucidate its role in CINV prophylaxis.

Cannabinoids

The combination of weak antiemetic efficacy with potentially beneficial side effects (sedation, euphoria) makes cannabinoids a useful adjunct to modern antiemetic therapy in selected patients. However, the associated side effects of dizziness and dysphoria should not be underestimated [6,14]. Cannabinoids are advised in patients intolerant of or refractory to 5-HT$_3$-RAs or steroids, and aprepitant [12,14]. Interestingly, in a systematic review of the efficacy of oral cannabinoids in the prevention of nausea and vomiting, it was found that cannabinoids were slightly better than conventional antiemetics (eg, metoclopramide, phenothiazines, haloperidol) [47]. Despite this, their clinical utility was found to be generally limited by the high incidence of adverse events, such as dizziness, dysphoria, and hallucinations [47,48].

Benzodiazepines

Benzodiazepines can be a useful additions to antiemetic regimens in certain circumstances. They are often used to treat anxiety and reduce the risk of anticipatory CINV. Benzodiazepines are also used in patients with refractory and breakthrough emesis [6,41].

Antihistamines

Antihistamines have been administered both as antiemetics and adjunctive agents to prevent dystonic reactions with dopamine antagonists [49]. Studies with diphenhydramine or hydroxyzine in the prevention of CINV have not shown that these drugs have antiemetic activity [19].

In palliative care, the antihistamines have a role in the treatment of nausea thought to be mediated by the vestibular system. Side effects of antihistamines include drowsiness, dry mouth, and blurred vision. Because of a lack of proven efficacy in several studies, antihistamines should not be utilized as antiemetic agents in the prevention of CINV [4]. Antihistamines may, however, be a useful drug in the treatment of nausea and vomiting when these symptoms are not induced by the chemotherapy itself [6].

Herbs as antiemetics

Herbs are used by at least 80% of the world's population and are increasingly popular. Some studies showed a potential benefit of ginger and peppermint in postoperative nausea and vomiting as well as in the management of nausea and vomiting in pregnancy.

Ginger (Zingiber officinale Roscoe)

The detailed mechanism of action of ginger is unknown, although it is known to exert its antiemetic effect at the gut and not at the central nervous system level [50]. Ginger is consumed via oral ingestion of powdered extract capsules in doses of 250–500 mg taken up to three times daily. The results of studies of the use of ginger by patients receiving chemotherapy are controversial [51,52]. However, at the ASCO meeting in 2009, Ryan et al suggested a superior effect of ginger versus placebo in terms of reducing nausea after emetogenic chemotherapy in 644 cancer patients [53].

Peppermint (Mentha x piperita Lamiaceae)

Peppermint acts as an internal calcium channel-blocking agent, producing intestinal smooth muscle relaxation. There is evidence supporting its use in patients with dyspepsia or irritable bowel syndrome and as an intraluminal spasmolytic agent during barium enemas and endoscopy [54]. There have been no published studies using peppermint as an adjunctive therapy for patients receiving chemotherapy. Peppermint seems to lessen this symptom in the treatment of postoperative nausea [55].

References

1   Hesketh PJ, Grunberg S, Gralla R, et al. The oral neurokinin-1 antagonist aprepitant for the prevention of chemotherapy-induced nausea and vomiting: a multinational, randomised, double-blind, placebo-controlled trial in patients receiving high-dose cisplatin. *J Clin Oncol.* 2003; 21: 4112-4119.
2   Jordan K, Sippel C, Schmoll HJ. Guidelines for antiemetic treatment of chemotherapy-induced nausea and vomiting: past, present, and future recommendations. *Oncologist.* 2007;12:1143-1150.
3   Poli-Bigelli S, Rodrigues-Pereira J, Carides AD, et al. Addition of the neurokinin 1 receptor antagonist aprepitant to standard antiemetic therapy improves control of

chemotherapyinduced nausea and vomiting. Results from a randomised, double-blind, placebo-controlled trial in Latin America. *Cancer*. 2003;97:3090-3098.

4 Hesketh PJ. Chemotherapy-induced nausea and vomiting. *N Engl J Med*. 2008;358:2482-2494.

5 Jordan K, Hinke A, Grothey A, Schmoll HJ. Granisetron versus tropisetron for prophylaxis of acute chemotherapy-induced emesis: a pooled analysis. *Support Care Cancer*. 2005;13:26-31.

6 Jordan K, Schmoll HJ, Aapro MS. Comparative activity of antiemetic drugs. *Crit Rev Oncol Hematol*. 2007;61:162-175.

7 Jordan K, Hinke A, Grothey A, et al. A meta-analysis comparing the efficacy of four 5-HT3 –receptor antagonists for acute chemotherapy-induced emesis. *Support Care Cancer*. 2007;15:1023-1033.

8 Rojas C, Thomas AG, Alt J, et al. Palonosetron triggers 5-HT(3) receptor internalization and causes prolonged inhibition of receptor function. *Eur J Pharmacol*. 2010; 626:193-199.

9 Rojas C, Li Y, Zhang J, et al. The antiemetic 5-HT 3 receptor antagonist palonosetron inhibits substance P-mediated responses in vitro and in vivo. *J Pharmacol Exp Ther*. 2010;335:362-368.

10 Navari RM. Palonosetron for the prevention of chemotherapy-induced nausea and vomiting in patients with cancer. *Future Oncol*. 2010; 6:1073-1084.

11 Ruhlmann C, Herrstedt J. Palonosetron hydrochloride for the prevention of chemotherapyinduced nausea and vomiting. *Expert Rev Anticancer Ther*. 2010;10:137-148.

12 Kris MG, Hesketh PJ, Somerfield MR, et al. American Society of Clinical Oncology guideline for antiemetics in oncology: update 2006. *J Clin Oncol*. 2006;24:2932-2947.

13 Roila F, Hesketh PJ, Herrstedt J. Prevention of chemotherapy- and radiotherapy-induced emesis: results of the 2004 Perugia International Antiemetic Consensus Conference. *Ann Oncol*. 2006;17:20-28.

14 Roila F, Herrstedt J, Aapro M, et al. Guideline update for MASCC and ESMO in the prevention of chemotherapy- and radiotherapy-induced nausea and vomiting: results of the Perugia consensus conference *Ann Oncol*. 2010:21(suppl 5):v232-v243.

15 Eisenberg P, Figueroa-Vadillo J, Zamora R, et al. Improved prevention of moderately emetogenic chemotherapy-induced nausea and vomiting with palonosetron, a pharmacologically novel 5-HT3 receptor antagonist: results of a phase III, single-dose trial versus dolasetron. *Cancer*. 2003;98:2473-2482.

16 Gralla R, Lichinitser M, Van Der Vegt S, et al. Palonosetron improves prevention of chemotherapyinduced nausea and vomiting following moderately emetogenic chemotherapy: results of a double-blind randomised phase III trial comparing single doses of palonosetron with ondansetron. *Ann Oncol*. 2003;14:1570-1577.

17 Saito M, Aogi K, Sekine I, et al. Palonosetron plus dexamethasone versus granisetron plus dexamethasone for prevention of nausea and vomiting during chemotherapy: a doubleblind, double-dummy, randomised, comparative phase III trial. *Lancet Oncol*. 2009;10:115-124.

18 Ettinger DS, Dwight D, MG K, eds. *National Comprehensive Cancer Network: Antiemesis, Clinical Practice Guidelines in Oncology*. Jenkintown, PA: National Comprehensive Cancer Network; 2005.

19 Gralla RJ, Osoba D, Kris MG, et al. Recommendations for the use of antiemetics: evidence-based, clinical practice guidelines. American Society of Clinical Oncology. *J Clin Oncol*. 1999;17:2971-2994.

20 Kris MG, Hesketh PJ, Herrstedt J, et al. Consensus proposals for the prevention of acute and delayed vomiting and nausea following high-emetic-risk chemotherapy. *Support Care Cancer*. 2005;13:85-96.

21 Goodin S, Cunningham R. 5-HT(3)-receptor antagonists for the treatment of nausea and vomiting: a reappraisal of their side-effect profile. *Oncologist*. 2002;7:424-436.

22 Grunberg SM. Antiemetic activity of corticosteroids in patients receiving cancer chemotherapy: dosing, efficacy, and tolerability analysis. *Ann Oncol*. 2007;18:233-240.

23 Aapro MS, Walko CM. Aprepitant: drug–drug interactions in perspective. *Ann Oncol*. 2010;21:2316-2323.

24 Italian Group for Antiemetic Research. Double-blind, dose-finding study of four intravenous doses of dexamethasone in the prevention of cisplatin-induced acute emesis. *J Clin Oncol.* 1998;16:2937-2942.

25 Italian Group for Antiemetic Research. Randomised, double-blind, dose-finding study of dexamethasone in preventing acute emesis induced by anthracyclines, carboplatin, or cyclophosphamide. *J Clin Oncol.* 2004;22:725-729.

26 Vardy J, Chiew KS, Galica J, et al. Side effects associated with the use of dexamethasone for prophylaxis of delayed emesis after moderately emetogenic chemotherapy. *Br J Cancer.* 2006;94:1011-1015.

27 Aapro M, Fabi A, Nolè F, et al. Double-blind, randomised, controlled study of the efficacy and tolerability of palonosetron plus dexamethasone for 1 day with or without dexamethasone on days 2 and 3 in the prevention of nausea and vomiting induced by moderately emetogenic chemotherapy. *Ann Oncol.* 2010;21:1083-1088.

28 Herr I, Ucur E, Herzer K, et al. Glucocorticoid cotreatment induces apoptosis resistance toward cancer therapy in carcinomas. *Cancer Res.* 2003;63:3112-3120.

29 Schmoll HJ, Aapro MS, Poli-Bigelli S, et al. Comparison of an aprepitant regimen with a multipleday ondansetron regimen, both with dexamethasone, for antiemetic efficacy in high-dose cisplatin treatment. *Ann Oncol.* 2006;17:1000-1006.

30 Rapoport B, Jordan K, Boice J, et al. Aprepitant for the prevention of chemotherapy-induced nausea and vomiting associated with a broad range of moderately emetogenic chemotherapies and tumor types: a randomised, double-blind study. *Support Care Cancer.* 2010;18:423-431.

31 Warr D, Grunberg, SM, Gralla, RJ, et al. The oral NK(1) antagonist aprepitant for the prevention of acute and delayed chemotherapy-induced nausea and vomiting: Pooled data from 2 randomised, double-blind, placebo controlled trials. *Eur J Cancer.* 2005; 41:1278-1285.

32 Chawla SP, Grunberg SM, Gralla RJ, et al. Establishing the dose of the oral NK1 antagonist aprepitant for the prevention of chemotherapy-induced nausea and vomiting. *Cancer.* 2003;97:2290-2300.

33 Grunberg SM, Chua DT, Maru A, et al. and the PN017 study group. Phase III randomized doubleblind study of single-dose fosaprepitant for prevention of cisplatin-induced nausea and vomiting. *J Clin Oncol.* 2010;28(suppl):Abstract 9021.

34 Depre M, Van Hecken A, Oeyen M, et al. Effect of aprepitant on the pharmacokinetics and pharmacodynamics of warfarin. *Eur J Clin Pharmacol.* 2005;61:341-346.

35 Shadle CR, Lee Y, Majumdar AK, et al. Evaluation of potential inductive effects of aprepitant on cytochrome P450 3A4 and 2C9 activity. *J Clin Pharmacol.* 2004;44:215-223.

36 Dando TM, Perry CM. Aprepitant: a review of its use in the prevention of chemotherapy-induced nausea and vomiting. *Drugs.* 2004;64:777-794.

37 Massaro AM, Lenz KL. Aprepitant: a novel antiemetic for chemotherapy-induced nausea and vomiting. *Ann Pharmacother.* 2005;39:77-85.

38 McCrea JB, Majumdar AK, Goldberg MR, et al. Effects of the neurokinin1 receptor antagonist aprepitant on the pharmacokinetics of dexamethasone and methylprednisolone. *Clin Pharmacol Ther.* 2003;74:17-24.

39 Nygren P, Hande K, Petty KJ, et al. Lack of effect of aprepitant on the pharmacokinetics of docetaxel in cancer patients. *Cancer Chemother Pharmacol.* 2005;55:609-616.

40 de Jonge M, Huitema A, Holtkamp M, et al. Aprepitant inhibits cyclophosphamide bioactivation and thiotepa metabolism. *Cancer Chemother Pharmacol.* 2005;56:370-378.

41 Lohr L. Chemotherapy-induced nausea and vomiting. *Cancer J.* 2008;14:85-93.

42 Kris MG, Gralla RJ, Tyson LB, et al. Controlling delayed vomiting: double-blind, randomised trial comparing placebo, dexamethasone alone, and metoclopramide plus dexamethasone in patients receiving cisplatin. *J Clin Oncol.* 1989;7:108-114.

43 Moreno I, Rosell R, Abad A, et al. Comparison of three protracted antiemetic regimens for the control of delayed emesis in cisplatin-treated patients. *Eur J Cancer.* 1992;28A:1344-1347.

44 Italian Group for Antiemetic Research. Ondansetron versus metoclopramide, both combined with dexamethasone, in the prevention of cisplatin-induced delayed emesis. *J Clin Oncol.* 1997;15:124-130.

45 Navari RM, Einhorn LH, Loehrer PJ Sr, et al. A phase II trial of olanzapine, dexamethasone, and palonosetron for the prevention of chemotherapy-induced nausea and vomiting: a Hoosier oncology group study. *Support Care Cancer.* 2007;15:1285-1291.

46 National Comprehensive Cancer Network. *Antiemesis, Clinical Practice Guidelines in Oncology.* Fort Washington, PA: National Comprehensive Cancer Network; 2010.

47 Tramer MR , Carroll D, Campbell FA et al. Cannabinoids for control of chemotherapy-induced nausea and vomiting: a quantitative systematic review. *BMJ.* 2001;323:16-21.

48 Radbruch L, Nauck F. Review of cannabinoids in the treatment of nausea and vomiting. *Schmerz.* 2004;18:306-310.

49 Kris MG, Gralla RJ, Clark RA, et al. Antiemetic control and prevention of side effects of anti-cancer therapy with lorazepam or diphenhydramine when used in combination with metoclopramide plus dexamethasone. A double-blind, randomised trial. *Cancer.* 1987;60:2816-2822.

50 Sharma SS, Gupta YK. Reversal of cisplatin-induced delay in gastric emptying in rats by ginger (Zingiber officinale). *J Ethnopharmacol.* 1998 62:49-55.

51 Dupuis LL, Nathan PC. Options for the prevention and management of acute chemotherapy-induced nausea and vomiting in children. *Paediatr Drugs.* 2003;5:597-613.

52 Manusirivithaya S, Sripramote M, Tangjitgamol S, et al. Antiemetic effect of ginger in gynecologic oncology patients receiving cisplatin. *Int J Gynecol Cancer.* 2004;14:1063-1069.

53 Ryan JL, Heckler C, Dakhil SR, et al. Ginger for chemotherapy-related nausea in cancer patients: A URCC CCOP randomised, double-blind, placebo-controlled clinical trial of 644 cancer patients. *J Clin Oncol.* 2009;27(suppl):15s.

54 Koretz RL, Rotblatt M. Complementary and alternative medicine in gastroenterology: the good, the bad, and the ugly. *Clin Gastroenterol Hepatol.* 2004;2:957-967.

55 Tate S. Peppermint oil: a treatment for postoperative nausea. *J Adv Nurs.* 1997;26:543-549.

Development of this chapter was supported by funding from Helsinn

Chapter 6

Antiemetic prophylaxis of chemotherapy-induced nausea and vomiting

Before chemotherapy, it is crucial to clearly define the optimal prophylactic antiemetic therapy for acute and delayed nausea and vomiting and to implement it from the beginning, since symptom-oriented therapy at a later stage is ineffective in most cases. This is important especially for the prophylaxis of delayed emesis.

First the emetogenic potential of the planned chemotherapy regimen needs to be established. The cytostatic agent with the highest emetogenic potential determines the emetogenicity of the whole chemotherapy; there is no cumulative effect when further cytostatic agents with lower emetogenicity are added [1,2].

For outpatients it is important to establish a written treatment plan for the prophylaxis of delayed emesis. The lowest fully effective once-daily dose for each antiemetic agent should be used. At equivalent doses and bioavailabilities, the oral and intravenous routes have similar efficacy and safety [1,3,4].

This chapter summarizes the antiemetic therapy schemes that are recommended for the prevention of acute and delayed nausea and vomiting, and it also considers the antiemetic potential of the chemotherapies. These schemes are based on the recent 2009 MASCC/ESMO guidelines. The recommended daily doses of antiemetics for acute (day 1) and delayed (from day 2 onwards) chemotherapy-induced nausea and vomiting (CINV) are shown in Figures 6.1 and 8.1 [2].

M. Aapro et al., *Prevention of Nausea and Vomiting in Cancer Patients*, 37
DOI: 10.1007/978-1-907673-58-0_6, © Springer Healthcare 2013

Antiemetic prophylaxis of chemotherapy-induced nausea and vomiting: 2009 MASCC/ESMO guidelines

Emetogenicity of chemotherapy	Acute phase (up to 24 h after chemotherapy)	Delayed phase (following the first 24 h to 5 days after chemotherapy)
High (>90%)	**5-HT$_3$-RA** Palonosetron 0.50 mg PO/0.25 mg IV Granisetron 2 mg PO/ 1 mg (0.01 mg/kg) IV Ondansetron 24 mg PO/ 8 mg (0.15 mg/kg) IV Tropisetron 5 mg PO/IV Dolasetron 100 mg PO* + **Dexamethasone** 12 mg p.o/IV + **Aprepitant** 125 mg PO or **Fosaprepitant** 150 mg IV	*Days 2–3:* **Dexamethasone** 8 mg + **Aprepitant** 80 mg PO (unless 150 mg IV fosaprepitant on day 1) *Day 4:* **Dexamethasone** 8 mg b.i.d.
Moderate (30–90%)	*1. AC chemotherapy:* **5-HT$_3$-RA** Palonosetron 0.50 mg PO/ 0.25 mg IV Granisetron 2 mg PO/1 mg (0.01 mg/kg) IV Ondansetron 16 mg PO (8 mg b.i.d.)/8 mg (0.15 mg/kg) IV Tropisetron 5 mg PO/IV Dolasetron 100 mg PO* + **Dexamethasone** 8 mg p.o/IV + **Aprepitant** 125 mg PO or **Fosaprepitant** 150 mg IV	*1. AC chemotherapy:* Days 2–3: **Aprepitant** 80 mg PO (unless 150 mg IV fosaprepitant on day 1)
	2. Non-AC MEC: **Palonosetron** 0.5 mg PO/0.25 mg IV + **Dexamethasone** 8 mg PO/IV	*2. Non-AC MEC:* Days 2–3: **Dexamethasone** 8 mg, or 4 mg b.i.d.
Low (10–30%)	**Dexamethasone** or **5-HT$_3$-RA** (see above) or **dopamine receptor antagonist**	No routine prophylaxis
Minimal (<10%)	No routine prophylaxis	No routine prophylaxis

Figure 6.1 Antiemetic prophylaxis of chemotherapy-induced nausea and vomiting: 2009 MASCC/ESMO guidelines. If the NK-1 receptor antagonist is not available for AC chemotherapy, palonosetron is the preferred 5-HT$_3$ receptor antagonist. *The injection form of dolasetron should no longer be used to prevent nausea and vomiting associated with CINV (www.fda.gov/drugs/drugsafety/ucm237081.htm). 5-HT$_3$, 5-hydroxytryptamine-3; AC, anthracycline (doxorubicin or epirubicin)+ cyclophosphamide; ESMO, European Society of Medical Oncology; MASCC, Multinational Association for Supportive Care in Cancer; NK-1, neurokinin-1; RA, receptor antagonist. Based on data from Roila et al [2], MASCC/ESMO [5], and product information leaflets.

Prevention of acute nausea and emesis (within the first 24 hours of chemotherapy treatment)

Highly emetogenic chemotherapy

Patients should be treated with a combination of a 5-hydroxytryptamine-3 receptor antagonist (5-HT$_3$-RA), a neurokinin-1(NK-1)-RA (aprepitant), and a corticosteroid.

Moderately emetogenic chemotherapy

Patients receiving a combination of anthracycline plus cyclophosphamide-based chemotherapy should be given a triple combination of a 5-HT$_3$-RA, a NK-1-RA (aprepitant), and a corticosteroid. If aprepitant is not available, women receiving a combination of anthracycline plus cyclophosphamide should receive a combination of palonosetron plus dexamethasone [2].

Patients undergoing other moderately emetogenic chemotherapy regimens should be given a combination of the 5-HT$_3$-RA palonosetron and the corticosteroid dexamethasone.

Low emetogenic chemotherapy

In patients receiving chemotherapy of low emetic risk, a single agent, such as a low dose of a corticosteroid, is effective. In principle 5-HT$_3$-RAs are not constituents of the prophylactic armamentarium. In this area, overtreatment has been observed in clinical practice but should be avoided; for example, a patient who is treated with paclitaxel does not need a 5-HT$_3$-RA routinely.

Minimally emetogenic chemotherapy

For patients treated with agents of minimal emetic risk, no antiemetic drug should be routinely administered before chemotherapy.

Prevention of delayed nausea and emesis (days 2–5 after chemotherapy)

Cisplatin, doxorubicin, and cyclophosphamide in particular cause long-lasting nausea and emesis. The presence of delayed emesis is often underestimated, with the consequence that no adequate preventive measures are taken.

Highly emetogenic chemotherapy

Routine prophylaxis should consist of a NK-1-RA (aprepitant) and a corticosteroid (Figure 6.1). The addition of a further 5-HT$_3$-RA is not necessary [6].

Moderately emetogenic chemotherapy

Aprepitant should be used to prevent delayed nausea and vomiting in patients with breast cancer receiving a combination of anthracycline plus cyclophosphamide treated with a combination of aprepitant (or fosaprepitant), a 5-HT$_3$-RA and dexamethasone to prevent acute nausea and vomiting. If these patients were not treated with a combination of aprepitant and a 5-HT$_3$-RA, but received palonosetron for the prevention of acute nausea and vomiting, dexamethasone treatment is preferred for the prevention of delayed nausea and vomiting.

In patients receiving chemotherapy of moderate emetic risk (which does not include a combination of anthracycline plus cyclophosphamide) in which palonosetron is recommended, multiday oral dexamethasone treatment is preferred for the prevention of delayed nausea and vomiting.

Low and minimally emetogenic chemotherapy

No routine prophylactic antiemetic treatment is planned for the delayed phase.

Therapy against anticipatory nausea and vomiting

The best approach to anticipatory nausea and vomiting (ANV) is to avoid the appearance of this phenomenon by using optimal antiemetic prophylaxis from the first cycle. ANV is a conditioned reflex, and drug therapy has modest efficacy. Conventional antiemetics are mostly ineffective for ANV and furthermore have not been extensively tested. Treatment with benzodiazepines in addition to conventional antiemetics has shown some efficacy, if given before the chemotherapy. However, since ANV is a learned conditioned reflex, it is best managed by psychological techniques, although this may not represent an easy solution in daily practice. Some possible interventions include muscle relaxation, systemic desensitization, hypnosis, and cognitive distraction [7].

Therapy in cases of insufficient antiemetic efficacy

If a patient presents with emesis despite the preventive measures preceding chemotherapy, it should first be checked that the patient received the antiemetics according to the guidelines. Further treatment steps in this case will be independent of the emetogenic potential of the chemotherapy. In general, a repetition of the previously given antiemetic agents usually does not produce the desired result. This is true particularly for first generation 5-HT$_3$-RAs [8,9]. It has been suggested that there is a better rationale for the addition of palonosetron as its mechanism of action may differ from other serotonin antagonists [10]. For patients who received a combination of a 5-HT$_3$-RA with a corticosteroid, a NK-1-RA (aprepitant) should be added. However, it has not yet been clarified whether the additional NK-1-RA has the ability to displace the already bound substance P from the receptor site on the NK-1 receptor [11].

With lasting emesis, the addition of metoclopramide, benzodiazepines, neuroleptic agents and in particular olanzapine may be effective [12]. The following drugs/dosages can be used with caution in frequently sedated patients:

- Metoclopramide: 10 mg IV or 20–40 mg PO every 4–6 hours;
- Olanzapine: one 5–10 mg tablet;
- Benzodiazepine: lorazepam one or two 1 mg tablets; alprazolam 0.25–1.0 mg tablet;
- Domperidone: 10–20 mg PO 3–4 times per day, maximum daily dose 80 mg;
- Haloperidol: 0.5–2 mg PO every 8–12 hours or 1–2 mg short IV infusion;
- Promethazine: 25–50 mg orally 3–4 times per day;
- Chlorpromazine: 25–50 mg slowly IV; and
- Dronabinol: 5–10 mg PO every 3–6 hours (maximum recommended daily dose 50 mg).

In addition, in parallel to pharmacological therapy, other causes of continuing emesis (such as emetogenic cotherapies, brain metastases, and gastrointestinal obstructions) should always be evaluated as potential etiological factors.

Multiday chemotherapy

For multiday cisplatin therapy, the use of a 5-HT$_3$-RA and a corticosteroid is recommended on the days when cisplatin is administered to the patients (acute phase). The ASCO guidelines recommend the same combination for multiple days of noncisplatin chemotherapy agents of high emetic risk [4,13]. In addition, for the prophylaxis of delayed CINV, on days 2 and 3 after chemotherapy, a corticosteroid alone should be administered. Aprepitant may be used for multi-day chemotherapy regimens that are likely to be highly emetogenic [14]. The MASCC/ESMO guidelines mention the use of a 5-HT$_3$ receptor antagonist on days 1–5, or palonosetron on days 1, 3, and 5 [2].

High-dose chemotherapy

There is a lack of studies in the high-dose chemotherapy setting. On the days when high-dose chemotherapy is administered (acute phase), the use of a 5-HT$_3$-RA and a corticosteroid is recommended before initiation of chemotherapy. On days 2 and 3 after high-dose chemotherapy, a corticosteroid alone should be given for the prevention of delayed CINV. The addition of a NK-1-RA to the 5-HT$_3$ receptor antagonist and corticosteroid, or the specific use of palonosetron as the 5-HT$_3$ receptor antagonist, can be taken into consideration, but it is not explicitly recommended by the recent guidelines.

References

1   Roila F, Hesketh PJ, Herrstedt J. Prevention of chemotherapy- and radiotherapy-induced emesis: results of the 2004 Perugia International Antiemetic Consensus Conference. *Ann Oncol*. 2006;17:20-28.

2   Roila F, Herrstedt J, Aapro M, et al. Guideline update for MASCC and ESMO in the prevention of chemotherapy- and radiotherapy-induced nausea and vomiting: results of the Perugia consensus conference *Ann Oncol*. 2010:21(suppl 5):v232-v243.

3   Jordan K, Bokemeyer C, Langenbrake C, Link H. Antiemetische Prophylaxe und Therapie gemas den MASCC und ASCO Guidelines: In: *Kurzgefasste interdisziplinare Leitlinien 2008 der Deutschen Krebsgesellschaft*. Munich, Germany: Zuckschwerdt Verlag; 2008:348-354.

4   Kris MG, Hesketh PJ, Somerfield MR, et al. American Society of Clinical Oncology guideline for antiemetics in oncology: update 2006. *J Clin Oncol*. 2006;24:2932-2947.

5   Multinational Association of Supportive Care in Cancer and European Society for Medical Oncology (ESMO). MASCC/ESMO Antiemetic Guidelines 2010. www.mascc.org/mc/page. do?sitePageId=88041. Accessed October 17, 2012.

6 Schmoll HJ, Aapro MS, Poli-Bigelli S, et al. Comparison of an aprepitant regimen with a multipleday ondansetron regimen, both with dexamethasone, for antiemetic efficacy in high-dose cisplatin treatment. *Ann Oncol.* 2006;17:1000-1006.

7 Aapro MS, Molassiotis A, Olver I. Anticipatory nausea and vomiting. *Support Care Cancer.* 2005;13:117-121.

8 Aapro MS. How do we manage patients with refractory or breakthrough emesis? *Support Care Cancer.* 2002;10:106-109.

9 Musso M, Scalone R, Crescimanno A, et al. Palonosetron and dexamethasone for prevention of nausea and vomiting in patients receiving high-dose chemotherapy with auto-SCT. *Bone Marrow Transplant.* 2010;45:123-127.

10 Einhorn LH, Grunberg SM, Rapoport B, et al. Antiemetic therapy for multiple-day chemotherapy and additional topics consisting of rescue antiemetics and high-dose chemotherapy with stem cell transplant: review and consensus statement. *Support Care Cancer.* 2011;19(suppl 1):S1-S4.

11 Jordan K. Neurokinin-1-receptor antagonists: a new approach in antiemetic therapy. *Onkologie.* 2006;29:39-43.

12 Hesketh PJ. Chemotherapy-induced nausea and vomiting. *N Engl J Med.* 2008;358:2482-2494.

13 Gralla RJ, Osoba D, Kris MG, et al. Recommendations for the use of antiemetics: evidence-based, clinical practice guidelines. American Society of Clinical Oncology. *J Clin Oncol.* 1999;17:2971-2974.

14 National Comprehensive Cancer Network. *Antiemesis, Clinical Practice Guidelines in Oncology.* Fort Washington, PA: National Comprehensive Cancer Network; 2010.

Development of this chapter was supported by funding from Helsinn

Chapter 7

Antiemetic prophylaxis of radiotherapy-induced nausea and vomiting

Although radiotherpy-induced nausea and vomiting (RINV) is often less severe than chemotherapy-induced nausea and vomiting (CINV), these side effects can be quite distressing. RINV is still often underestimated by radiation oncologists. However, as many as 50–80% of patients undergoing radiotherapy will experience these side effects, depending on the site of irradiation. The traditional management of RINV has been empirical, using non-specific antiemetic agents. Progress in understanding the pathophysiology and treatment of chemotherapy-induced emesis has enhanced our understanding of RINV. Although the pathophysiology of RINV is incompletely understood, it is thought to be similar to that caused by chemotherapy (see Chapter 2).

Uncontrolled nausea and vomiting may result in patients delaying or refusing further radiotherapy. The incidence and severity of nausea and vomiting depend on radiotherapy-related factors (irradiated site, single and total dose, fractionation, irradiated volume, radiotherapy techniques) and on patient-related factors (gender, general health of the patient, age, concurrent or recent chemotherapy, psychological state, tumor stage).

The guideline proposed at MASCC/ESMO in 2009 [1,2] will be summarized in this chapter.

M. Aapro et al., *Prevention of Nausea and Vomiting in Cancer Patients*,
DOI: 10.1007/978-1-907673-58-0_7, © Springer Healthcare 2013

Antiemetics and their efficacy for radiotherapy-induced nausea and vomiting

Only a few small randomized clinical trials have evaluated the efficacy of various antiemetic drugs in preventing RINV. Generally, patients entering these trials are those receiving total body irradiation (TBI), half body irradiation (HBI) or upper-abdomen irradiation because of the higher risk of developing nausea and/or vomiting. Evidence suggests that preventative treatment is better than intervention on an as-needed basis.

Serotonin receptor antagonists

In the last decade, the 5-hydroxytryptamine-3 receptor antagonists (5-HT$_3$-RAs) have been used more extensively to treat RINV in clinical practice [3]. Figures 7.1 and 7.2 show randomized trials with 5-HT$_3$-RAs and/or corticosteroids in patients submitted to radiotherapy with single or fractionated regimens. Different compounds and a wide range of doses and schedules have been used.

The seven published trials, mostly studying ondansetron in patients submitted to upper-abdomen irradiation, showed that 5-HT$_3$-RAs achieved significantly greater protection against RINV than did metoclopramide, phenothiazines, or placebo [4–9] (Figure 7.1). Also, in patients treated with TBI or HBI, 5-HT$_3$-RAs provided significantly better protection for RINV than placebo or conventional antiemetics, as expected [12–17] (Figure 7.2).

Side effects were evaluated and compared by Goodin and Cunningham [18]. The adverse effects of 5-HT$_3$-RAs were generally mild, with headache, constipation, diarrhea, and asthenia being most common [9,12,14,19]. Sometimes, rather than causing constipation, 5-HT$_3$-RAs reduced the frequency of diarrhea, a troublesome side effect due to acute enteric radiation toxicity [6,20].

The relatively new 5-HT$_3$-RA palonosetron and the transdermal granisetron patch might be an interesting option, especially for patients receiving radiotherapy. To date, only a few abstracts have become available on the use of palonosetron and the transdermal granisetron patch in RINV, showing promising activity [21–24].

Randomized clinical trials with 5-HT₃ receptor antagonists and/or steroids in patients undergoing upper abdomen irradiation

Study	n	Radiotherapy regimen	Antiemetic treatment	Complete response (% of patients)	Result
Priestman et al [8]	154	≥5 fractions to minimum total dose of 20 Gy	DEX 2 mg × 3/day PO for 5–7 days	70	DEX better than placebo
			Placebo	49	
Bey et al [5]	50	≥6 Gy single fraction	DOL 0.3 mg/kg IV	100*	DOL better than placebo
			DOL 0.6 mg/kg IV	93*	
			DOL 1.2 mg/kg IV	83*	
			Placebo	54*	
Lanciano et al [7]	260	10–30 fractions (1.8–3 Gy/fraction)	GRAN 2 mg/day	57.5	GRAN better than placebo
			Placebo	42	
Priestman et al [8]	82	8–10 Gy single fraction	OND 8 mg × 3/day PO for 5 days	97	OND better than PCP
			PCP 10 mg × 3/day PO for 5 days	46	
Priestman et al [9]	135	1.8 Gy/day for at least 5 fractions	OND 8 mg × 3/day PO	61	OND better than MCP (for vomiting)
			MCP 10 mg × 3/day PO	35	
Franzen et al [6]	111	≥1.7 Gy/day for ≥10 fractions	OND 8 mg × 2/day PO	67	OND better than placebo
			Placebo	45	
Wong et al [10]	211	≥15 fractions to the upper abdomen to a dose of 20 or more Gy	OND 8 mg bid for 5 days + placebo for 5 days	71† 12‡	OND + DEX better than OND alone
			OND 8 mg bid + DEX 4 mg for 5 days	78† 23‡	
Aass et al [4]	23	2 Gy/day to 30 Gy in 15 fractions	TRO 5 mg/day PO	91	TRO better than MCP
			MCP 10 mg × 3/day PO	50	
Mystakidou et al [11]	288	Fractionated radiotherapy of moderate or high emetogenic potential	5 mg TRO daily starting 1 day before radiotherapy until 7 days after end of radiotherapy 5 mg TRO on an as needed basis	Incidence of vomiting was 2.19 times higher in the rescue TRO arm (P=0.001)	Prophylactic TRO better than rescue TRO

Figure 7.1 **Randomized clinical trials with 5-HT₃ receptor antagonists and/or steroids in patients undergoing upper abdomen irradiation.** *Complete plus major response. †Primary end point: complete response during days 1–5. ‡Secondary end point: complete response during days 1–15. DEX, dexamethasone; DOL, dolasetron; GRAN, granisetron; MCP, metoclopramide; OND, ondansetron; PCP, prochlorperazine; TRO, tropisetron. Adapted from Feyer et al [1].

Randomized clinical trials with 5-HT₃ receptor antagonists in patients undergoing total-body irradiation and half-body irradiation

Study	n	Radiotherapy regimen	Antiemetic treatment	Complete response (% of patients)	Result
Prentice et al [12]	30	7.5 Gy TBI single fraction	GRAN 3 mg IV versus	53	GRAN better than MTC + DEX + LOR
			MTC 20 mg IV + DEX 6 mg/m² IV + LOR 2 mg IV	13	
Tiley et al [16]	20	10.5 Gy TBI single fraction	OND 8 mg IV	90*	OND better than placebo
			Placebo	50*	
Spitzer et al [13]	20	1.2 Gy × 3/day TBI 11 fractions to a total dose of 13.2 Gy	OND 8 mg × 3/day PO	50	OND better than placebo
			Placebo	0	
Sykes et al [15]	66	8–12.5 Gy HBI single fraction	OND 8 mg × 2 PO versus	34	OND better than CLP + DEX
			CLP 25 mg × 3 PO + DEX 6 mg × 3 PO		
Huang et al [17]	116	7–7.7 Gy	OND 8 mg (IV) + DEX 10 mg versus	84	OND + DEX better than paspertin + DEX
			MTC 10 mg + DEX 10 mg	20	
Spitzer et al [14]	34	1.2 Gy × 3/day TBI 11 fractions to a total dose of 13.2 Gy	OND 8 mg × 3/day PO versus	47	No difference
			GRAN 2 mg × 1/day PO	61	

Figure 7.2 Randomized clinical trials with 5-HT₃ receptor antagonists in patients undergoing total-body irradiation and half-body irradiation. *All patients received IV dexamethasone (8 mg) and phenobarbitone (60 mg/m²). CLP, chlorpromazine; CR, complete response; DEX, dexamethasone; GRAN, granisetron; LOR, lorazepam; MTC, metoclopramide; OND, ondansetron. Adapted from Feyer et al [1].

Corticosteroids

Their widespread availability, low-cost, and recorded benefit make corticosteroids very attarractive antiemetic drugs. One double-blind study has been published to date examining the use of dexamethasone as a single agent for the prophylaxis of RINV [23]. Patients who underwent fractionated radiotherapy to the upper abdomen received either oral dexamethasone (2 mg three times daily) or placebo only in the first week of radiotherapy, even though the courses lasted up to 6 weeks (Figure 7.1).

The effect of adding a short course of low-dose dexamethasone (days 1–5) to a 5-HT$_3$-RA was assessed in a National Cancer Institute of Canada trial, in which 211 patients receiving radiotherapy to the upper abdomen were studied [10] (see Figure 7.1). During the first 5 days, there was a nonsignificant trend toward improved complete control of nausea (50% vs 38 % with placebo) and vomiting (78% vs 71%) (ie, primary end point was not reached). However, the effects of dexamethasone extended beyond the initial period: significantly more patients had complete control of emesis over the entire course of radiotherapy (23% vs 12%, with placebo) (ie, secondary end point was reached). Although this study did not demonstrate a statistically significant benefit for the primary end point, results on several secondary end points as well as quality-of-life data strongly suggest that benefits do exist with the addition of dexamethasone.

Considering that the majority of emetic episodes occur early in the treatment course, it is indeed arguable that prophylactic antiemetics may not be necessary for a full course of radiotherapy and therefore treatment for the first week might be sufficient [23–25].

Neurokinin-1 receptor antagonists

Extensive clinical trials have established an important role for the NK-1-RAs in the management of CINV [26]. Aprepitant has not been formally tested for patients with RINV in randomized trials, and therefore it cannot be recommended, even though the pathogenesis of RINV is thought to be mediated in part by substance P [27].

Other agents

Older, less specific antiemetic drugs such as prochlorperazine, metoclopramide, and cannabinoids have shown limited efficacy in the prevention or treatment of RINV, although they may retain a role in patients with milder symptoms. Cannabinoids have been no more effective than the dopamine antagonists and showed an inferior safety profile, including sedation and euphoria/dysphoria.

Duration of prophylaxis

The appropriate duration of 5-HT$_3$-RA prophylaxis for patients receiving fractionated radiotherapy is not clear. Although randomized trials have used 5-HT$_3$-RAs either for extended periods [6,8,10] or just for the first five treatments, there have been no randomized trials that compare these approaches. The decision on whether to continue prophylactic treatment beyond the first week should be based upon an assessment of the risk of emesis as well as other relevant individual factors.

Rescue therapy

The beneficial role of 5-HT$_3$-RAs as rescue medication has been suggested in all conducted trials [11,28,29]. The role of rescue medication should be further explored in the setting of low and minimal risk of RINV because the incidence of nausea and vomiting in the moderate and high emetogenic risk group is rather high and prophylactic use of antiemetics is mandatory in this setting.

Guideline-based prophylaxis and treatment of radiotherapy-induced nausea and vomiting

The development of new agents to treat chemotherapy-induced emesis and clinical trials in patients with RINV have led to improvements in the control of RINV. The 5-HT$_3$-RAs and corticosteroids are the most extensively evaluated agents in patients with RINV. These advances are incorporated into the 2009 MASCC/ESMO guidelines for antiemetic prophylaxis and treatment [1,2].

According to the irradiated area (the most frequently studied risk factor), the guidelines are divided into four risk-levels: high, moderate, low, and minimal emetogenic risk of radiotherapy [1]. The updated guidelines are shown in Figure 7.3.

- **High risk:** TBI is associated with a high risk of RINV. In patients receiving TBI, prophylaxis with a 5-HT$_3$-RA is recommended.

Radiotherapy-induced emesis: radiation emetic risk levels and new MASCC and ESMO recommendations

Risk level	Risk factors	Antiemetic guidelines	MASCC evidence (level of scientific confidence/level of consensus)	ESMO evidence (type of evidence/grade of recommendation)
High	TBI	Prophylaxis with 5-HT$_3$-RA + DEX	High/high (For the addition of DEX: moderate/high)	II/B (For the addition of DEX: IIIC)
Moderate	Upper abdomen, HBI, UBI	Prophylaxis with 5-HT$_3$-RA + optional DEX	High/high (For the addition of DEX: moderate/high)	II/A (For the addition of DEX: IIB)
Low	Cranium (all), craniospinal, head and neck, lower thorax region, pelvis	Prophylaxis or rescue with 5-HT$_3$-RA	Moderate/high For rescue: low/high	III/B For rescue: IV/C
Minimal	Extremities, breast	Rescue with dopamine receptor antagonist or 5-HT$_3$-RA	Low/high	IV/D

Figure 7.3 Radiotherapy-induced emesis: radiation emetic risk levels and new MASCC and ESMO recommendations. *In concomitant radiochemotherapy the antiemetic prophylaxis is according to the chemotherapy-related antiemetic guidelines of the corresponding risk category, unless the risk of emesis is higher with radiotherapy than chemotherapy. 5-HT$_3$-RA, 5-HT$_3$ receptor antagonist; DEX, dexamethasone; HBI, half body irradiation; TBI, total body irradiation; UBI, upper body irradiation. Based on data from Feyer et al [1].

The addition of dexamethasone to the 5-HT$_3$-RAs has not been formally studied. However, if this approach adds efficacy, as occurs with chemotherapy, such a regimen would be appropriate for patients undergoing TBI.

- **Moderate risk:** radiation of the upper abdomen, HBI and UBI is associated with a moderate risk of RINV. In patients receiving radiotherapy with moderate emetogenic risk, prophylaxis with a 5-HT$_3$-RA and optionally in combination with a short course (day 1–5) of dexamethasone is recommended.

- **Low risk:** radiation of the cranium (all), craniospinal region, head and neck, lower thorax region and pelvis is associated with a low risk of RINV. In patients receiving radiotherapy with low emetogenic risk, prophylaxis or a rescue therapy with a 5-HT$_3$-RA is suggested.

- **Minimal risk:** radiation of the extremities and breast is associated with a minimal risk of RINV. In patients receiving radiotherapy with low emetogenic risk, rescue with a dopamine-RA or prophylaxis with a 5-HT$_3$-RA is recommended.
- **Concomitant chemotherapy:** in patients undergoing concomitant radiochemotherapy, antiemetic prophylaxis should be according to the the emetogenic risk category of the used chemotherapeutic regimen defined by the CINV guidelines. In cases in which the risk category of radiotherapy is higher than the concomitant chemotherapy, the antiemetic treatment should be tailored accordingly to the risk category of radiotherapy.

References

1   Feyer P, Maranzano M, Molassiotis A, et al. Radiotherapy-induced nausea and vomiting (RINV): MASCC/ESMO Guideline for Antiemetics in Radiotherapy: update 2009. *Support Care Cancer.* 2011(suppl 1):S5-S14.

2   Roila F, Herrstedt J, Aapro M, et al. Guideline update for MASCC and ESMO in the prevention of chemotherapy- and radiotherapy-induced nausea and vomiting: results of the Perugia consensus conference *Ann Oncol.* 2010:21(suppl 5):v232–v243.

3   Feyer P, Seegenschmiedt MH, Steingraeber M. Granisetron in the control of radiotherapy-induced nausea and vomiting: a comparison with other antiemetic therapies. *Support Care Cancer.* 2005;13:671-678.

4   Aass N, Hatun DE, Thoresen M, Fossa SD. Prophylactic use of tropisetron or metoclopramide during adjuvant abdominal radiotherapy of seminoma stage I: a randomised, open trial in 23 patients. *Radiother Oncol.* 1997;45:125-128.

5   Bey P, Wilkinson PM, Resbeut M, et al. A double-blind, placebo-controlled trial of i.v. dolasetron mesilate in the prevention of radiotherapy-induced nausea and vomiting in cancer patients. *Support Care Cancer.* 1996;4:378-383.

6   Franzen L, Nyman J, Hagberg H, et al. A randomised placebo controlled study with ondansetron in patients undergoing fractionated radiotherapy. *Ann Oncol.* 1996;7:587-592.

7   Lanciano R, Sherman DM, Michalski J, et al. The efficacy and safety of once-daily Kytril (granisetron hydrochloride) tablets in the prophylaxis of nausea and emesis following fractionated upper abdominal radiotherapy. *Cancer Invest.* 2001;19:763-772.

8   Priestman TJ, Roberts JT, Lucraft H, et al. Results of a randomised, double-blind comparative study of ondansetron and metoclopramide in the prevention of nausea and vomiting following high-dose upper abdominal irradiation. *Clin Oncol (R Coll Radiol).* 1990;2:71-75.

9   Priestman TJ, Roberts JT, Upadhyaya BK. A prospective randomised double-blind trial comparing ondansetron versus prochlorperazine for the prevention of nausea and vomiting in patients undergoing fractionated radiotherapy. *Clin Oncol (R Coll Radiol).* 1993;5:358-363.

10 Wong RK, Paul N, Ding K, et al. 5-hydroxytryptamine-3 receptor antagonist with or without shortcourse dexamethasone in the prophylaxis of radiation induced emesis: a placebo-controlled randomised trial of the National Cancer Institute of Canada Clinical Trials Group (SC19). *J Clin Oncol.* 2006;24:3458-3464.

11 Mystakidou K, Katsouda E, Linou A, et al. Prophylactic tropisetron versus rescue tropisetron in fractionated radiotherapy to moderate or high emetogenic areas: a prospective randomized open label study in cancer patients. *Med Oncol.* 2006;23:251-262.

12 Prentice HG, Cunningham S, Gandhi L, et al. Granisetron in the prevention of irradiation-induced emesis. *Bone Marrow Transplant*. 1995;15:445-458.

13 Spitzer TR, Bryson JC, Cirenza E, et al. Randomised double-blind, placebo-controlled evaluation of oral ondansetron in the prevention of nausea and vomiting associated with fractionated total body irradiation. *J Clin Oncol*. 1994;12:2432-2438.

14 Spitzer TR , Friedman CJ, Bushnell W, et al. Double-blind, randomised, parallel-group study on the efficacy and safety of oral granisetron and oral ondansetron in the prophylaxis of nausea and vomiting in patients receiving hyperfractionated total body irradiation. *Bone Marrow Transplant*. 2000;26:203-210.

15 Sykes AJ, Kiltie AE, Stewart AL. Ondansetron versus a chlorpromazine and dexamethasone combination for the prevention of nausea and vomiting: a prospective, randomised study to assess efficacy, cost effectiveness and quality of life following single-fraction radiotherapy. *Support Care Cancer*. 1997;5:500-503.

16 Tiley C, Powles R, Catalano J, et al. Results of a double blind placebo controlled study of ondansetron as an antiemetic during total body irradiation in patients undergoing bone marrow transplantation. *Leuk Lymphoma*. 1992;7:317-321.

17 Huang X, Guo N, Fan Y. [Ondansetron in the prophylaxis of acute emesis induced by supra-high single dose total body irradiation (TBI)]. *Zhonghua Zhong Liu Za Zhi*. 1995;17:64-66.

18 Goodin S, Cunningham R. 5-HT(3)-receptor antagonists for the treatment of nausea and vomiting: a reappraisal of their side-effect profile. *Oncologist*. 2002;7:424-436.

19 Jordan K, Schmoll HJ, Aapro MS. Comparative activity of antiemetic drugs. *Crit Rev Oncol Hematol*. 2007;61:162-175.

20 Feyer PC , Stewart AL, Titlbach OJ. Aetiology and prevention of emesis induced by radiotherapy. *Support Care Cancer*. 1998;6:253-260.

21 Belli C, Dahl T, Herrstedt J. Palonosetron plus prednisolone in patients receiving fractionated radiotherapy plus weekly cisplatin. *Support Care Cancer*. 2008;16:01-004.

22 Dimitrijevic J, Medic-Milijic N. Prevention of nausea and vomiting induced by chemotherapy followed by combined chemo/radiotherapy in head and neck cancer patients. *Support Care Cancer*. 2009;17:02-009.

23 Kirkbride P, Bezjak A, Pater J, et al. Dexamethasone for the prophylaxis of radiation-induced emesis: a National Cancer Institute of Canada Clinical Trials Group phase III study. *J Clin Oncol*. 2000;18:1960-1966.

24 Feyer P, Maranzano E, Molassiotis A, et al. Radiotherapy-induced nausea and vomiting (RINV): antiemetic guidelines. *Support Care Cancer*. 2005;13:122-128.

25 Kris MG, Hesketh PJ, Somerfield MR, et al. American Society of Clinical Oncology guideline for antiemetics in oncology: update 2006. *J Clin Oncol*. 2006;24:2932-2947.

26 Jordan K, Schmoll HJ, Aapro MS. Comparative activity of antiemetic drugs. *Crit Rev Oncol Hematol*. 2007; 61:162-175.

27 Yamamoto K, Nohara K, Furuya T, Yamatodani A. Ondansetron, dexamethasone and an NK 1 antagonist block radiation sickness in mice. *Pharmacol Biochem Behav*. 2005;82:24-29.

28 LeBourgeois JP, McKenna CJ, Coster B, et al. Efficacy of an ondansetron orally disintegrating tablet: a novel oral formulation of this 5-HT(3) receptor antagonist in the treatment of fractionated radiotherapy-induced nausea and emesis. Emesis Study Group for the Ondansetron Orally Disintegrating Tablet in Radiotherapy Treatment. *Clin Oncol (R Coll Radiol)*. 1999;11:340-347.

29 Maranzano E, Feyer P, Molassiotis A, et al. Evidence-based recommendations for the use of antiemetics in radiotherapy. *Radiother Oncol*. 2005;76:227-233.

Development of this chapter was supported by funding from Helsinn

Summary of the approach to treatment of chemotherapy-induced nausea and vomiting

We conclude with a summary to help plan antiemetic prophylaxis in the setting of daily practice:

- Establish the emetogenic potential of the chemotherapy (see Figures 3.1 and 3.2).
    - The chemotherapeutic agent with the highest emetogenic potential determines the emetogenic level of the whole therapy.
    - There is no cumulative effect in combination therapies.
- Prophylactic antiemetic treatment is crucial. It is important to note that the appearance of delayed emesis is often underestimated; consequently, the prophylaxis for days 2–5 has to be thought out in advance, with well-planned prophylaxis instituted from the beginning.
- Antiemetic prophylaxis is summarized in Figure 8.1, as shown on page 48.
- For persisting chemotherapy-induced nausea and vomiting there is also a necessity to consider possible differential diagnosis (eg, brain metastases).

Additional details of guideline recommendations can be found at the following web sites:

- www.mascc.org
- www.esmo.org
- www.nccn.org
- www.asco.org

M. Aapro et al., *Prevention of Nausea and Vomiting in Cancer Patients*, DOI: 10.1007/978-1-907673-58-0_8, © Springer Healthcare 2013

Antiemetic prophylaxis of chemotherapy-induced nausea and vomiting: 2009 MASCC/ESMO guidelines

Emetogenicity of chemotherapy	Acute phase (up to 24 h after chemotherapy)	Delayed phase (following the first 24 h to 5 days after chemotherapy)
High (>90%)	**5-HT$_3$-RA** Palonosetron 0.50 mg PO/ 0.25 mg IV	*Days 2–3:* **Dexamethasone** 8 mg + **Aprepitant** 80 mg PO (unless 150 mg IV fosaprepitant on day 1)
	Granisetron 2 mg PO/ 1 mg (0.01 mg/kg) IV	
	Ondansetron 24 mg PO/ 8 mg (0.15 mg/kg) IV	
	Tropisetron 5 mg PO/IV	
	Dolasetron 100 mg PO* + **Dexamethasone** 12 mg p.o/IV +	
	Aprepitant 125 mg PO or **Fosaprepitant** 150 mg IV	*Day 4:* **Dexamethasone** 8 mg b.i.d.
Moderate (30–90%)	*1. AC chemotherapy:* **5-HT$_3$-RA** Palonosetron 0.50 mg PO/ 0.25 mg IV	*1. AC chemotherapy:* *Days 2–3:* **Aprepitant** 80 mg PO (unless 150 mg IV fosaprepitant on day 1)
	Granisetron 2 mg PO/ 1 mg (0.01 mg/kg) IV	
	Ondansetron 16 mg PO (8 mg b.i.d.)/ 8 mg (0.15 mg/kg) IV	
	Tropisetron 5 mg PO/IV	
	Dolasetron 100 mg PO* + **Dexamethasone** 8 mg p.o/IV + **Aprepitant** 125 mg PO or **Fosaprepitant** 150 mg IV	

Figure 8.1 Antiemetic prophylaxis of chemotherapy-induced nausea and vomiting: 2009 MASCC/ESMO guidelines (continues overleaf).

Antiemetic prophylaxis of chemotherapy-induced nausea and vomiting: 2009 MASCC/ESMO guidelines (continued)

Emetogenicity of chemotherapy	Acute phase (up to 24 h after chemotherapy)	Delayed phase (following the first 24 h to 5 days after chemotherapy)
	2. Non-AC MEC:	*2. Non-AC MEC:*
	Palonosetron 0.50 mg p.o/ 0.25 mg IV + **Dexamethasone** 8 mg p.o/IV	Days 2–3: **Dexamethasone** 8 mg, or 4 mg b.i.d.
Low (10–30%)	**Dexamethasone** or **5-HT$_3$-RA** (see above) or **dopamine receptor antagonist**	No routine prophylaxis
Minimal (<10%)	No routine prophylaxis	No routine prophylaxis

Figure 8.1 Antiemetic prophylaxis of chemotherapy-induced nausea and vomiting: 2009 MASCC/ESMO guidelines (continued). If the NK1 receptor antagonist is not available for AC chemotherapy, palonosetron is the preferred 5-HT$_3$ receptor antagonist. *The injection form of dolasetron should no longer be used to prevent nausea and vomiting associated with CINV (http://www.fda.gov/drugs/drugsafety/ucm237081.htm). 5-HT$_3$-RA, 5-hydroxytryptamine-3 receptor antagonist; AC, anthracycline (doxorubicin or epirubicin)+ cyclophosphamide; ESMO, European Society of Medical Oncology; MASCC, Multinational Association for Supportive Care in Cancer; MEC, moderately emetogenic chemotherapy; NK-1, neurokinin-1. Based on data from MASCC/ESMO [1], Roila et al [2], and product information leaflets.

References

1   Multinational Association of Supportive Care in Cancer and European Society for Medical Oncology (ESMO). MASCC/ESMO Antiemetic Guidelines 2010. www.mascc.org/mc/page.do?sitePageId=88041. Accessed October 17, 2012.
2   Roila F, Herrstedt J, Aapro M, et al. Guideline update for MASCC and ESMO in the prevention of chemotherapy- and radiotherapy-induced nausea and vomiting: results of the Perugia consensus conference *Ann Oncol*. 2010:21(suppl 5):v232-v243.

Development of this chapter was supported by funding from Helsinn

Chapter 9

Conclusions and future directions

Progress in the control of nausea and vomiting related to cancer therapy has been remarkable. However, many questions remain open, and not all patients are adequately protected against cancer therapy-induced nausea and vomiting.

We lack randomized studies investigating whether palonosetron, in combination with a neurokinin-1-receptor antagonist (NK-1-RA), should be preferred over the other 5-hydroxytryptamine-3 receptor antagonists due to its contribution to the prevention of delayed chemotherapy-induced nausea and vomiting, and we hope that this will be addressed in the future. We also look forward to the development of other NK-1-RAs.

We need better guidance for the treatment of patients who, after optimal preventative treatment, nevertheless experience nausea and vomiting. In the delayed phase, emerging studies indicate that dexamethasone-sparing regimens might be an option and this strategy should be further investigated. However, it remains the best drug for delayed nausea, which is a challenge.

Nausea is a subjective phenomenon which is understood in different ways and not easily measured. We should remain aware that it is likely that for patients, this term encompasses many different reasons for being unwell after chemotherapy.

M. Aapro et al., *Prevention of Nausea and Vomiting in Cancer Patients*,
DOI: 10.1007/978-1-907673-58-0_9, © Springer Healthcare 2013